Cancer Dance

By Catherine McClain

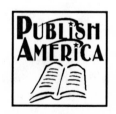

PublishAmerica
Baltimore

ISBN:1-60441-730-7
PUBLISHED BY PUBLISHAMERICA, LLLP
www.publishamerica.com
Baltimore

Printed in the United States of America

A gift for you!

TO: _____

FROM: _____

~*~*~*~*~*~*~*~*~*~*~*~*~

_____

_____

_____

_____

_____

_____

This book is dedicated to my Mom
for her unconditional love,
immeasurable grace,
and endless support.

Acknowledgments

The following acknowledgements may be a bit too sappy for most of you to read. I have always been an optimistic, upbeat personality (drives some people nuts). You may not be as blessed to be surrounded by this amount of love and support. For that, I wish you better. As for me, these thank yous do not even begin to express my appreciation for those listed here (and those I forget to mention). If this is too much love for you to handle, you can skip right over to the beginning of the book.

I recognize that I could never have made it through my cancer experience without the love and support of family and friends…and a few strangers. Most of all, I came to understand and appreciate the importance of thanking the Spiritual Universe on a daily basis. I have never considered myself a religious person (raised Catholic) but I always considered myself spiritual. I wasn't. I am now. My first thank you goes to the God within me.

I'd like to thank the members of the academy, yadda, yadda, yadda. Not! My mother and father not only provided me with love and encouragement during my cancer experience, they have done that my entire life. They predisposed me to the positive attitude that made this journey a blessing. My second thank you goes to my wonderful parents. I always feel surrounded by their love.

I can't figure out who to put next in line. My son Paul has been in my life longer than Charlie (Charlie was my fiancé at the time of my cancer and my husband for a short time afterward). But, I don't want either of them to feel slighted because I thanked one of them before the other. So, my third thank you goes to both of the men who were in my life at the time of these writings, in that order. Now, I will go alphabetically to further elaborate on the grace they provide for me.

Charlie put up with me through my toughest time. Enough said. That is not an easy task, and for that alone, he deserves an award. Not only was he by my side through the entire cancer experience, he even married me when I was going through my Tamoxifen rages. Perhaps he is a little masochistic, but he is certainly one of the most incredible loving men I have ever known.

Paul, my son, is one of the greatest human beings on the planet. For a young adult, he has the wisdom of a sage, a kind heart, and an open mind. He never even went through the terrible twos (I'm afraid to see what his 40's will be like). I can't take full credit for him turning out so well, as a single parent, my village of loving friends and family helped him become who he is today. He also comes from good genes, as his father (my first husband), is one of those kind and loving men as well.

My fourth thank you goes to my guardian angels; Carol, Lisla, Sheila, Olivia, Michelle and Mo. This is my supportive circle of co-workers who where there for me from the moment I received the diagnosis phone call from my doctor until today. I received never ending words of encouragement, offers of help, and spiritual support. Thank you too Tommy for teaching me the miracle of prayer and the value of faith (hanging in there, no matter what the circumstance).

My next thank you goes to my Bosom Buddies (other breast cancer survivors) who taught me some wonderful coping strategies for getting through treatment. We communicated mostly through e-mail (my virtual support group) but their advice and encouragement was better than medicine. Thank you mom, Phyllis, Betty, Susan, Missy, Joyce, and Linda… just to name a few.

I am blessed to be surrounded by some wonderful friends (or should I say, I choose to surround myself with wonderful people). Although I did not spend as much time with my friends during my journey as I would have liked, their constant connection to me via e-mail and the phone broadened my circle of healing light. Thank you Joe, Heather, John, Greg, Ruth, Leslie (Fug), David, Sue, Nana, Pam, Pam and Pam, Catherine, Edward, Kimberly Amber, Kimber, Nantz, Jan, Katie, cousin Sandy and all the others I forgot to mention. A special thank you to Joan, a woman I hardly know. You will read some of her messages to me in this book and will then understand how she has touched my life. A huge thank you to Steve Peterson for reviewing my book and helping me develop my writing skills with advice and recommended readings.

Thank you to the American Cancer Society, the Susan G. Komen Foundation, Dr. Susan Love, all my doctors and nurses (especially SES) and all the people who have chosen to work in this profession and to do cancer research. A special thank you to Jim and Trish for making the Surviving Beautifully Fashion Show such an incredible annual event that changes people's lives.

And last but not least, thank you to every one who asked to receive my e-mail updates and encouraged me to keep writing. The synergy we experienced by me sharing with you (and your replies) created this book. I hope I have given you as much as you have given me as we celebrate life, one day at a time.

Namaste!

Table of Contents

A Day in the Office 13

Setting the Stage 14

Cathy Updates

6/22/02—Cathy Update #1
10 Days After Diagnosis 19

6/28/02—Cathy Update #2
2 Weeks Since Diagnosis 22

7/7/02—Cathy Update #3
Prep Week: Count Down to Surgery 25

7/8/02—Day of Surgery 31

7/9/02—Cathy Update #4
Post-Surgery Update 35

7/12/02—Cathy Update #5
Two Steps Forward Then One Step Back 36

7/18/02—Cathy Update #6
"Listen to Your Body" 40

7/23/02—Cathy Update #7
It's Not About the Breast 44

7/27/02—Cathy Update #8
It's Not About the Hair 47

7/31/02—Update #9
Cathy Shares Reply 50

8/4/02—Cathy Update #10
Hello Dolly 54

7/28/02–8/1/02 California Youth Leadership
Forum for Students with Disabilities 59

8/11/02—Cathy Update #11
AB FAB and Pill Stuff 62

8/13/02—Cathy Update #12
First AC Treatment 64

8/18/02—Cathy Update #13
Blowin' in the Wind 68

8/26/02—Cathy Update #14
Hair Today, Gone Tomorrow 73

9/2/02—Cathy Update #15
Cathy's Glamour Tips 78

9/8/02—Cathy Update #16
Working the Arm 83

9/15/02—Cathy Update #17
I'm Fine 88

9/22/02—Cathy Update #18
The Benefits of Benefits 89

9/30/02—Cathy Update #19
Fried Eggs and Toast 92

10/7/02—Cathy Update #20
Dare to Dream 96

10/13/02—Cathy Update #21
The Grapes of Wrath 99

10/21/02—Cathy Update #22
Mirror, Mirror on the Wall 102

10/27/02—Cathy Update #23
The Long and Winding Road 107

11/3/02—Cathy Update #24
Trick or Treat 110

11/10/02—Cathy Update #25
Taxotere…Tax of Tears 113

11/17/02—Cathy Update #26
Mowf Pobems 116

11/25/02—Cathy Update #27
Ob-la-di, Ob-la-da 120

12/01/02—Cathy Update #28
Gobble, Gobble 123

12/9/02—Cathy Update #29
It's the Pits 127

12/15/02—Cathy Update #30
What Goes Up, Must Come Down 129

12/22/02—Cathy Update #31
Traditions 131

12/29/02—Cathy Update #32
Ode to a Dad 134

1/7/03—Cathy Update #33
Happy New Year 138

1/19/03—Cathy Update #34
Clowns to the Left of Me 141

1/29/03—Cathy Update #35
Michael Update 144

2/3/03—Cathy Update #36
Let It Be 145

2/13/03—Cathy Update #37
Radiation 147

3/3/03—Cathy Update #38
Two Weeks More 151

3/4/03—Cathy Update #39
Paul Update 154

3/13/03—Cathy Update #40
Hallelujah 155

4/10/03—Cathy Update #41
Pack and Purge 158

4/18/03—Cathy Update #42
Surviving Beautifully 161

5/5/03—Cathy Update #43
Feliz Cinco de Mayo 164

5/18/03—Cathy Update #44
Relay for Life 167

6/12/03—Cathy Update #45
Final Update, One Year Post Diagnosis 171

My Charmed Life 173

Epilogue 179

A Day in the Office...

...just like any other. I spent the morning running from one meeting to another interpreting for a couple of my deaf clients. Change is in the air as the recent reorganization of my department continues to confuse us. I still didn't know who to ask questions of and trust that I was going to get an accurate answer. My secretary Carol and I were in her office discussing (or should I say, disgusting) our views of just how frustrating the recent turn of events has been. Managers are being moved around like pieces in a chess game. Who knows who will be our new boss and will we like the new chain of command? Uncertainty can be so unsettling.

The phone line to my office lights up on Carol's console and I pick it up and press the button to connect to the incoming call.

"Cathy McClain," I answer. It is my surgeon calling from his office. He has the results of my biopsy.

Just a few days earlier I had been to his office for a needle core biopsy of a suspicious lump in my left breast. Damn, those biopsies hurt! I was still feeling a bit sore from it since he took 10 core samples from my lump. Ouch! I wasn't too worried though. I had a suspicious cyst removed from my right breast 17 years earlier and it turned out to be nothing. I expected the same results this time around.

"Your biopsy results showed malignancy," he said. He wanted me to come to his office right away and discuss my options. I couldn't believe my ears. How could this be? How could he tell me over the phone? How am I going to get home? How, why, where, when? I was in shock.

Somehow I managed to maintain my composure as I ended the phone call and hung up. I turned to Carol and told her, "I have cancer" and ran down the hall to my office. She followed in close pursuit. There in my office she held me as I cried.

This Is My Story

Setting the Stage

This book is a compilation of e-mail messages I sent to my co-workers, friends and family as I was going through breast cancer treatments. I compiled the book two years after my diagnosis and this publication occurred 2 years later. The initial updates are geared toward an audience of people who knew me well enough to not need much explaining. Eventually more people asked to receive my updates, some of whom I didn't know, but by that time they had become quite familiar with me. You (the reader of this book) don't know me from Adam (which Adam do they mean? Adam, Eve's partner? Adam West? Adam Sandler?) So, I write this section for you to better understand these updates. Also, if you can't handle optimism in large doses, I recommend you read this book one update at a time. I've always seen the positive side of life, and some pessimists struggle to comprehend. They are, however, the ones who need to be exposed to optimism more often. This book is for those who need that boost to endure life's ups and downs and for those who are encountering their own cancer diagnosis or that of a loved one.

Disclaimer

This is my story. Don't try this at home. It does not reflect the experience of all who have had cancer. I am not a medical expert, so don't consider the medical information here to be always accurate. It is only my understanding of what I learned about my treatment. I attempt to apply my sense of humor throughout my writing. This is not intended to disrespect the seriousness of this topic. I choose to laugh in the face of cancer. I choose to laugh every day. You are welcome to laugh with me, but please don't hold it against me if you don't find it funny. (Some of my humor isn't funny, but more silly, or sarcastic, or stupid)

You MAY have a similar experience as mine if you happen to be a 41 year old woman of Portuguese, Scottish, English, Irish decent. If you are 5' 2" tall, in good physical condition (except for the cancer). If you have one son, a supportive family and a good employer, comfortable wages with excellent medical and disability benefits (less stress). If you have skilled physicians, caring nurses and loving friends. If all of these conditions exist, and you happen to be diagnosed with the exact same type of tumor I had, then maybe, just maybe, your experience will be the same as mine. Otherwise, just glean from this book what ever you find helpful, whether or not you ever have cancer. The point I am trying to make in this book is....LIVE, LAUGH, LOVE!! No matter how much more time you have (or don't have) on this planet. Live each day to the fullest.

The Stage

I am a sign language interpreter. In American Sign Language, before telling a story, we spatially set up the "stage" of the environment we are going to describe, then move each character from here to there to provide a 3 dimensional representation of the experience we are sharing. It's very effective, so I'm going to do the same here for you.

At the time I wrote these updates, my home and work were in different towns. My home town was Tracy, and my fiancé Charlie lived in Paradise over 80 miles away. Although my original diagnosis was in Tracy, I chose to have surgery in Sacramento (and I had my chemotherapy and radiation treatments in Stockton (30 miles away).

Cast of Characters

At the time I wrote these updates, my name was Catherine McClain (thus the initials at the end of each update "cMc"). I was the Disabilities Services Program manager for a large employer, providing accommodation services to employees with disabilities. In this job I also did sign language interpreting, my first passion and profession. I was a single mother of a 17 year old son (Paul) at the time of diagnosis and I was engaged for 4 years to Charlie.

My initial audience of readers was co-workers, family and friends. They started sending my updates to their friends and family, so by the last update, I had an e-mail list of over 150 people. Who knows how many people eventually read them. Some of the names have been changed in this book to protect people's privacy. The silly names of the doctors are actually what I called them during my treatment (OK, perhaps not to their face, except for Papa Smurf).

Chatty Cathy

Do you remember the doll that was popular in the 1960's, Chatty Cathy? Pull the string on the back of her neck and she talked. (High tech for those times). I have always lived up to that name, never lacking for words, and getting in trouble for talking in school. I make fast friends with strangers on airplanes and trains (some who are still close friends today). I'm never shy about sharing personal information. My life is an open book. I never considered writing for pleasure, but discovered over the course of these e-mails, I love to write.

My intention in writing updates to my family and friends was to avoid talking about my cancer every time I saw someone. If I send the cancer information out in an e-mail, they will have all the details, and we can focus on pleasant conversation and not dwell repeatedly on the cancer subject. The more I wrote, the more I enjoyed writing. This is obvious as you see the updates getting longer as time goes by. It developed into a tool to educate people about cancer. Then it became an avenue for me to journal my deepest thoughts and feelings (therapy for my recovery). You will notice at the end of the early updates, I provide a post script giving people permission to share the information with others. Because of privacy laws, it is illegal in the work place (and now everywhere) to share medical information about people. Since many of my original audience was co-workers, I wanted to provide permission to share the information, so no one got in trouble.

In the process of my recovery from surgery, I was also recovering from a fast paced obsessive compulsive lifestyle. Many of my revelations are regarding my need to slow down and approach life differently. This is just as much a journal of spiritual recovery and reevaluating my life and lifestyle as it is a cancer journal.

Why Publish?

Why not? I admit it would be nice for me to earn enough money to pay for my son's college, however I am not about money. Much of the proceeds from the sales of this book will go toward several Disability and Cancer related non-profit organizations and events you'll read about. The Youth Leadership Forum, Media Access Awards and scholarships for students with disabilities are fantastic programs that are in danger of ending because they are primarily state funded. I would also like to provide support to the American Cancer Society's Relay for Life and St. Joseph's Cancer Center Surviving Beautifully fashion show. Both of these cancer events had an incredibly positive impact on my recovery. Through the course of my cancer journey, I have realized that the more I give, the more I am rewarded. Nothing would please me more than to offer support to organizations who are struggling because other people don't have the opportunity to give enough.

I didn't plan to publish, but so many people encouraged me to do so, who am I to deny God's confirmations. Some people told me that reading my updates gave them a spiritual uplift. Cancer patients told me that reading my updates helped them with their own treatment struggles. Some told me they learned a lot about cancer and now better understand what their mother, father, uncle, cousin, etc. went through. If just one person's life is better for having read this, then it is all worth it.

My purpose in publishing this book is to provide cancer patients with a virtual support group of two (themselves and me); to somehow ease their path in this icky journey; to see the positive side of life during a difficult time. My purpose is to help loved ones understand the inner feelings of cancer patients who are not able to express what is inside. My purpose is to educate people about breast cancer (well, at least the kind I had) and hopefully encourage women to take charge of their health before cancer strikes. My purpose is to say "Hey, don't wait until you get cancer to realize your spiritual potential."

You will notice several writing styles in my updates. Most of the information between parenthesis ( ) are my snide remarks or attempts at being funny. Some of them just add more information. Anything small remarks you see in *italics* have been added while I edited this book to provide hind sight (picture a butt with bifocals). The text in *italics* is not part of my original updates. In my original updates I sited several song lyrics, as in most of our lives, music sings our story. Due to copyright laws, I did not include entire song lyrics in this book, however you can better understand where I am coming from if you look up the lyrics. So if you see the words (sing along) and you know the tune, please sing while you read it (out loud if you want). You may also notice that the beginning updates are mostly educational, and my writing is a bit unpolished. I was a novice. I am hoping that my writing improved as the updates continued and that the reader will become more engaged as the updates unfold.

Book Title

I had a tough time deciding what to title the book. My original thought was "Cathy Updates" since basically that is what this is (Too boring). Then, I thought I should add the ever popular colon phrase (talking grammar, not intestines), "Cathy Updates: My Breast Cancer Journey" (Blahhhh!). Then the spiritual nature of my experience came to me, and I thought about "Cathy Updates: My Cancer Induced Awakening" (Too academic). Then the humor starting coming out as I wanted to select something catchy. People don't read what they don't notice. So these titles came to mind; "Cathy's Cancer Trip," "Das Boob," "My Left Tit," "It's About the Hair," "Help me, My Turban's too Tight," and "My Trip Down Mammary Lane." One thing I did learn on this journey…I can't force something to be. Time provides all answers, and so it did with finding the right title.

One aspect of my life that consistently keeps me moving, dreaming and creating is my love of signing to music and my love of dance. For years I have performed many sign/song presentations for various celebratory events. It's always been a dream of mine to sign a song alive on stage with Melissa Etheridge (my favorite artist and a sister breast cancer survivor). Most recently I've incorporated sign into my belly dance performances. Although I didn't feel like physically dancing through much of my journey, I never forgot to "dance" through my experience. As I was going through my updates and compiling them for publication, this theme rang louder. At that time I had recently performed a signed song interpretation at that year's Surviving Beautifully Fashion Show, a fundraiser for St. Joseph's Cancer Center and an uplifting experience for cancer patients. The song so beautifully sung by Trish was titled "I Hope you Dance" (lyrics by Mark Sanders and Tia Sillers, well known as performed by Lee Ann Womack). If you've ever heard this song and listened carefully to the lyrics, it really sums up my purpose for publishing this book. So, that is when I decided to title the book "Cancer Dance."

I hope this book is as much of a gift to you as you are to me for reading it.

I hope you dance!

Cathy Updates

6/22/02—Cathy Update #1
(10 Days After Diagnosis)

This is the first of several updates to give you a status report of "Cathy's Cancer Trip." Please don't be offended by the humor I throw in every now and then. I am actually quite OK with this and it seems to be bothering others more than me. You have my permission to share this info with others.

I'm either lying on the beach in Encinitas or pottery shopping in Tecate Mexico as you read this. What?! How can she do that? Isn't she supposed to be miserable? Why hasn't she had surgery yet? Is she crazy? Those of you who have known me a while know the answer to that last question. YES. Crazy, but not stupid. I have seen several doctors and had several tests already. I am now waiting for my appointment with the surgeon I have chosen. That will be Wednesday June 26. Meanwhile, Charlie and I had this vacation planned already, so why not go and enjoy my last chance to shake loose for many months. Contrary to popular belief, there is no hurry.

Dr. Susan Love's Breast Book (3rd edition) is an excellent resource for breast cancer information. It is my main text book as I research surgical and treatment methods. If you have boobs, get this book. She covers every aspect of breast care, not just cancer. According to Dr. Love, at this stage I have already had this cancer for more than 5 years. Taking the time to get the treatment I believe in with a surgeon that I trust is more important than rushing to the operating table.

Breast cancer runs in both sides of my family, so I have been watching my fibrocystic breasts for many years. (I guess some men have too) In 1984 I had a surgical biopsy on a lump that blocked my milk ducts as I was breast feeding. This was simply a benign cyst. One year later, my mother was diagnosed with the exact same cancer I have. She had a modified radical mastectomy, chemotherapy and hormone therapy. She is healthy to this day, and by my side as I go through this.

I have been watching this recent lump fairly closely for the past year. My last 3 mammograms were only 6 months apart. The problem with fibrocystic breasts is they don't mammogram clearly. Everything looks suspicious, even healthy tissue. I have my new gynecologist to thank for insisting that an ultra sound be done. She isn't familiar with my lumps and when I went for my annual "female" exam, she didn't like the way the lump felt. I was used to it, so I wasn't worried (I had an evaluation by a surgeon a year before who told me, "that doesn't look like anything suspicious. I don't think we need to biopsy it." Looking back, I wish I had insisted he did). The ultra sound was suspicious. The lump did not have a uniform shape like a cyst. May 15 was my ultra sound, June 10 was my needle core biopsy, June 12 I received my diagnosis. I have invasive ductal breast cancer (the most popular type). Fortunately, it is a slow growing form of cancer. Prior to my biopsy, the tumor was 1.2 cm (as measured by the ultra sound). Now, after 8 needle core samples were removed, I don't know what size it is. We won't know whether or not I have Stage I or Stage II cancer until after the lymph node(s) under my arm are evaluated during my surgery (Stage I means the tumor is smaller than 2 cm and has not spread. Stage II is a tumor larger than 2 cm or one that has spread outside the original tumor). I had a bone scan on June 21 and my bones appear to be clear of any cancer.

Since the removal of my lymph nodes can lead to Lymphedema (swelling of the arm), I want to avoid losing too many of them. As a sign language interpreter, I don't know if I could still interpret if I developed this condition that limits arm movement. However, we won't know if the cancer has spread to my lymphatic system unless the nodes are evaluated. For this reason, I have chosen to participate in a new clinical trial being conducted at my Cancer Center in Sacramento. The Sentinel Node Biopsy procedure offers the chance to evaluate only one or two lymph nodes and possibly avoid removing any others. In this surgery, a dye is injected into the tumor and the doctor watches to see which lymph node that tumor drains to. This is the sentinel node. The probability that cancer has spread to this node first before any others is very high. If that node is dissected and tested for cancer, and there is none there, then no more lymph nodes are removed. If cancer is found in the sentinel node, then all my lymph nodes will be removed and many of them examined. (major bummer)

Since my tumor size is so small, I have opted for a lumpectomy and radiation therapy instead of a mastectomy without radiation. I don't like the idea of radiation therapy, but I am quite fond of my nipple and would like to keep it. Some say the younger you are, the more aggressive the cancer is. For this reason, chemotherapy is recommended. Some people may disagree with this theory. All I know is there is a 30% chance that the chemotherapy will prevent the cancer from becoming active in other parts of my body in case it has already spread. Seeing that the life expectancy of metastasized breast cancer is less than 5 years, I don't want to take any chances. Knowing the history of cancer in my family, I would rather lose my hair than take any chances of losing my life. At this time, I am choosing to do chemotherapy.

Many questions are still unanswered and I will know more after my appointment with the surgeon on June 26. By then I should know if I qualify to participate in the clinical study. I will know my surgery date. As I learn more, I will let you know.

I have already received so, so many wonderful cards and messages from my friends and family. I feel totally supported (and maybe a little smothered) but considering the "C" word is involved, it feels good to do an inventory of all the lives I get to share in. Life is good, and I plan to enjoy every last minute of it.

Thank you for being there for me. I will send another update after my appointment with the surgeon.

Love, hugs and smooches to all of you.

cMc

6/28/02—Cathy Update #2
(2 Weeks Since Diagnosis)

It has been so wonderful to hear from so many of you. I have people from all religions praying for me. That should mean I am covered in every corner of heaven. I am so fortunate, wealthy in my friendships. Thank you all so much for making this ordeal so full of hope and love.

After my peaceful R&R in Encinitas California (not Encinada Mexico, as some of you thought, but far more beautiful) I hit the road running upon my return. I had an appointment with my oncologist Wednesday morning in Stockton and discussed chemotherapy options. We won't make decisions until after the tumor and lymph node are evaluated, but the popular course of action these days seems to be AC (Adriamycin and Cytoxan) with a possible follow up of Taxol. (there is a chemistry quiz at the end of this e-mail, so pay attention) My mother received CMF treatments in 1984 (Cytoxan, methotrexate and 5-fluorouracil) and did not lose her hair and I was hoping to follow the same course of action hoping to receive the same benefit of saving my hair. Alas, that was 16 years ago and much has been learned since then. Today AC has a bad rap as being a very harsh treatment. The oncologist says it is now given in lower doses than before, so it shouldn't be a problem. One way to avoid problems with my veins reacting to the chemical is to have a port and catheter inserted into my chest so I won't be poked dozens of times in the arm with needles for blood tests and chemo treatments. I will probably choose this method as my arms are precious to my career (and hugging my nieces).

Wednesday afternoon I met my surgeon in Sacramento at Sutter Cancer Center. I call him Papa Smurf (remember the cartoon?). He was wearing Smurf colored scrubs and stands well above 6 feet tall. (anything over 5'9" is tall to me) What a sweetheart, and better yet, extremely experienced in the Sentinel Node biopsy procedure. I will be receiving this procedure for my surgery, however I will not be participating in the clinical trial. The trial involves selecting patients at random to have the Sentinel Node biopsy, then other patients will have Sentinel node and other nodes evaluated too. I don't want to take the chance of not being a single node donor, so I am not going to participate in the trial. I apologize to future breast cancer patients for my selfish decision. As a sign language interpreter, I just can't risk getting lymphodema.

As excited as I was to learn that I will be getting the surgery I chose from the surgeon I selected, my balloon soon burst when I heard the surgery date…July 16. My heart sank. For the first time since I heard of my diagnosis, I could feel depression setting in as the day wore on. That would be 36 days after my biopsy. My tumor is so close to my lymph nodes already and the biopsy did a lot of destruction, I was so worried that would be too long to wait. Worried the cancer would certainly spread. The next day I was e-chatting with a sister-survivor who informed me of some statistics regarding the timing of surgery. Having surgery within 28 days of biopsy appears to be the timing for greatest success. Encouraged by her info, I sent a fax to my Cancer Center explaining my concerns and mentioning the 28 day window. Papa Smurf came through for me. The next day I received a call from his office. My surgery was moved up to July 8, exactly 28 days post-biopsy. It will be at 6:00 pm, evidently Smurfs work overtime. I know, it is only 8 days difference, but those were going to be the longest 8 days of my life. Thank you Susan! (The moral of this story is… take charge of your medical treatment and don't be afraid to ask for what you believe in.)

So, I have one more week of work…shhhhhhh, don't tell anyone. I need to pack up my office because they are moving my office while I am gone. I don't want anyone to know I will be at work or else they will expect me to……do some work.

I head up to Charlie's (my fiancé) Paradise home Sunday July 7 (at this time I lived in Tracy, more than 80 miles away, and Charlie's home is closer to my surgeon in Sacramento). I have outpatient surgery on Monday July 8, and recover for one week in Paradise. If my lymph node shows signs of cancer, I will go back into surgery a few days later to have the rest of my lymph nodes removed. (this is the prayer part) I return to Tracy approximately one week after surgery and begin chemo treatments out of Stockton soon after.

If you would like to shower me with gifts, you can send them to Charlie's home. Otherwise, e-mail messages are absolutely cherished.

More e-mail updates after surgery.

Chemo Quiz

Now for the quiz and survey....

Quiz:

1. What type of chemotherapy treatment did Cathy's oncologist recommend? CMF, AC, or AC/DC
2. Who is Cathy's favorite surgeon? a. Papa Murphy b. Papa Smurf c. Papa Pill

Survey:

Cathy is wigging out. What color hair would you like to see her in? brown, dark brown, black, blonde, gray, red, platinum, wavy gravy

p.s. you have my permission to share this with others

7/7/02—Cathy Update #3
(1 day before lumpectomy and
Sentinal node biopsy surgery)

Prep Week: Count Down to Surgery

WOW, what a week. I have always known I am anal retentive and obsessive compulsive about planning, but this week takes the cake. One good thing (believe it or not) about the delay between diagnosis and surgery is having time to get all my ducks in a row, which in turn, will reduce my stress post-surgery (fortunately having a slow growing cancer gave me more time). My mom had her mastectomy 3 days after diagnosis (16 years ago). I have had 25 days to finish work related projects, delegate to others, learn more about BC (breast cancer) treatment options, communicate with other BC survivors, get 'supplies' in preparation for surgery, buy the books I have wanted to read but never had the time, and have FUN,FUN,FUN. Yes, that's right, the 3 letter word that starts with FU-. (that is three!! letters) There have been a few days when it caught up with me and I cried, for maybe 5 minutes or so, but I have lived such a full and enjoyable life since my diagnosis I haven't had time nor felt like getting depressed. I followed through with all of my original plans I made pre-diagnosis and spent time in the presence of wonderful family and friends who have showered me with joy. I'm keeping my fingers crossed that some of this glee will stay with me post-surgery.

The following is a run-down of events that have kept my spirits up and helped me feel prepared and able to face the inevitable. I highly recommend to anyone facing a cancer journey to stay engaged in life and remain as active as possible. It speeds the healing!

Three days after my diagnosis, one of my best friends (Leslie, a.k.a., Fug) and I went to the Fillmore in S.F. to see Davy Jones and Mickey Dolenz of the Monkees. How can that not be fun? (by the way, my a.k.a. is McFug) (Mickey was my favorite Monkee, but Davy has matured VERY well)

Five days post-diagnosis my former work group (I prefer to refer to them as my work-family) had a farewell party. We are undergoing a 'separation' due to a business reorganization. I have worked with some of these folks for 14 years and it was a wonderful celebration of our time together. When we got up to dance to Motown in the restaurant, others watched in envy (a facial expression that closely resembles "they're crazy.") For the first time since the beginning of my cancer journey, I didn't care what other people thought of me. (*a sentiment that lingers to this day*)

That evening I flew off to Las Vegas to interpret for an all-day meeting the next day at Nellis AFB. It meant a lot to me to be able to go since this job required two interpreters with top secret level security clearances and there were only two of us this side of the Mississippi available for that day. Yes, it was business, but we managed to visit the Venetian casino and shops before we flew home that night. What a place… incredible shops, gondola's with singing gondola-operators (do they have a word for that?), and a wonderful meal sitting under the false sky in an Italian courtyard. I felt like we were in the movie "Truman (you know, Jim Carey movie where he lives his while life on a movie set and doesn't know it)." I have always wanted to go there. (Venice, that is)

Three days later Charlie and I headed south for a brief visit with my good friend Ruth in L.A. and then off on vacation to Encinitas (not Encinada) for 4 days. Strolls on the beach, playing in the ocean, walks in the canyon, pottery shopping in Tecate Mexico and the company of wonderful friends. Need I say more.

Four days later I saw many family members at our annual Family Reunion, "The Portugues Picnic." (I am part Portagee and proud of it!) If you don't have a family reunion in your family, start one! It's times like this that we come to realize the importance of family. Don't wait until you get hurt or sick to find out you really love those crazy relatives. I spent a majority of my time at the reunion running around playing with my two-year old-niece. At times, I prefer to stay at that maturity level. She and I can really relate. (mentally, not just genetically)

On the drive back home, I stopped at the bookstore and bought books about cancer and nutrition. I want to learn about foods that may help reduce the negative side effects of chemo and also boost my immune system.

This past week began with the realization that no matter how much fun I am having, internally the stress is there. My neck and shoulders are constantly stiff, I am exhausted by 8:00 pm and I don't sleep as soundly as I usually do. I made sure that I planned massage therapy into my schedule as often as possible. I am a true believer that a good massage on a regular basis is imperative to overall health. If your work place has chair massage... DO IT! If not, find a massage therapist you trust. It has incredible healing powers.

Monday night I had my monthly full-body massage appointment with Joe, my massage therapist for the past 4 years. He is not only a great massage therapist, but also has a degree in Kinestheology (is that a word?) and is a 25 year cancer survivor. I asked him advice about vitamin and mineral supplements to help boost my immune system during chemo treatments. He also recommended I read the book by Lance Armstrong, "It's Not About the Bike" to learn Lance's perspective on how he faced his cancer. Joe is not only a helpful resource, he is an incredible spiritual human being and a dear friend. (You too Heather!)

Tuesday began with a chest x-ray to see if there is any sign of cancer spreading to my lungs. The most common places for Breast Cancer to spread to is the bones, lungs, liver and brain. My bones, lungs and liver all check out OK. My brain, well those who know me already know the answer to that one.—For lunch I met with a fellow employee who had BC surgery and treatment 3 years ago. She provided me with great advice about what to expect and helpful hints, (i.e. get pajamas and clothes that button down the front because it's hard to move your arm post-surgery). She also gave me 4 wigs, two hats and a few scarves. She recommended I join a support group as statistics show that women who participate in them have a greater survival rate.

Thanks B.B.—Later that evening I went shopping for new button front pajamas and tops.

Wednesday started with blood tests to evaluate my clotting factor before surgery. I have avoided all aspirin, ibuprofen products and high doses of vitamin E to avoid thinning of my blood which can cause excess bleeding during surgery.—Then a stop at the bookstore again to get Lance Armstrong's book and another one that may be helpful, "Meditation for Dummies" by Stephan Bodian (Gotta reduce this subconscious stress).—For lunch my mom and I went wig shopping at a wonderful breast cancer boutique in Pleasanton. This shop specializes in products for BC clients (bras, swim suits, prosthetics, scarves, wigs, etc.) and what a great staff. Jennifer had picked out a wig for me (since I stopped by briefly last week) that was PERFECT. It's going to be hard getting used to me with short hair, but I now own 5 wigs, so perhaps Murphy's Law will kick in and I won't lose the hair (wish, wish, hope, hope). The vote for my new hair color has leaned toward auburn/red (and puce), but unfortunately this manufacturer doesn't have auburn as an option and red is just going to make me more wild (can't have that). At 3:00 I had a half hour chair massage with Vickie. At 4:00 I went to the dentist to get my teeth cleaned. I had my appointment moved up a month because it is recommended to avoid the dentist while on chemo.

The risk of infection is higher and the gums and teeth are prone to bleeding and decay. I received special extra-fluoride toothpaste and was cautioned to brush after every meal and rinse with alcohol-free mouthwash to avoid irritating my gums. One thing I noticed about this day was that my pain tolerance level was very low. The blood draw was painful, as was the teeth cleaning. I don't usually feel pain during these procedures. Interesting. I wonder if anxiety is making more aware of pain.

Thursday was the 4th of July. Every year we go to Modesto for the Mayflower Court block party complete with 4 swimming pools, parade, frozen margaritas flow all day, talent show and fire works. This year for the talent show, my son Paul, my bud Fug, Charlie and I re-enacted Steve Martin's Saturday Night Live "King Tut" musical skit, complete with costumes. What a blast! Working toward this by sewing costumes and rehearsing was important to keep me focused on fun. I have been planning to do this skit since last year. I didn't want to miss it…and I didn't.

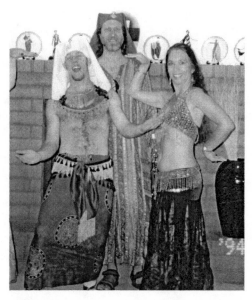

Oh so serious just 4 days before surgery.

Friday was my last day of work before my surgery. For my "last lunch" we were wiggin' out on sushi. Several of my co-workers brought in sushi and we all wore wigs for lunch. I brought the 4 that were given to me on Tuesday, plus 3 others I borrowed from Fug's talent show supply. This helped me to overcome my anxiety about wearing a wig to work when I return and hopefully will relieve my co-worker's apprehensionas well. Not to mention it was great fun. By the way, the wigs are still in my office if you want to stop by and try one on. At 2:20 I had a half hour chair massage. At the end of the work day, three of my favorite co-workers stood with me in prayer. Now, I am not one for formal prayer. I am surprised each time I enter a church and it isn't struck by lightening. I was so touched by the offer to do a prayer for me I wanted to join in. We all stood facing each other holding hands. As they prayed for me to find peace, I could feel the tears that had begun to flow stop and an overwhelming sense of peace came over me. Maybe there is something to this prayer stuff. I think I'll practice it more often. Thank you Tommy! You are a treasure in my life. After work I had the chance to visit with my friend Richard and his son Christopher from Mississippi. I haven't seen them in years and it was an extra treat that they were in town for the week so I could visit them while I still feel good.

So I am writing this as I pack up my stuff for my surgery followed by one week at Charlie's house. I am sad that my son Paul has to work all week and will not be by my side while I recover from surgery, but I believe it is best. He will have enough "reality" facing him when I am back home in Tracyand while I am going through treatments. I don't want to burden him with the boredom of being away from his life in Tracy. He is 17, almost 18 and this is an opportunity to learn to do the bachelor thing for a week. Stay tuned for future updates to discover how this works out. Hopefully, there won't be stories of empty beer bottles and undies on the lamp (He's a good boy, really… no really!).

Sorry this was so long. I've been busy, too busy to get scared. I have a lot of trust in my doctors and modern medical science. It is, by the way, the "marvel" of modern medicine. I don't like the phrase, the "miracle" of modern medicine because miracles are not man-made. I put my trust in my surgeon Papa Smurf; I put my faith in the power that overcame me during that prayer on Friday; and I put my love in all of you who are sending support my way.

More info post-surgery.

Love,

cMc

p.s. You have my permission to share… yadda, yadda, yadda.

7/8/02—Day of Surgery

This entry in the book was not one of my updates. I never did get around to writing about the day of my surgery, so here I am, 21 months later, reviewing notes from my journal and trying to remember the details of that day.

One of my clearest memories, and regrets, was my stubborn independent demeanor when checking into the hospital. Although Charlie and I had been engaged for several years, I have lived most of my adult life (and childhood for that matter) being fiercely independent. I wasn't acting like a fiancé. Part of me wanted to be alone and didn't want anyone around. I also know how sensitive Charlie is and I didn't want the pre-op process to cause him undue worry. Seeing the helplessness in his face was almost impossible to bear. I did not allow him to sit with me pre-op or "bother me" in post-op. How naive I was. I now realize that regardless of my feelings of independence, Charlie needed to be with me at this time. Even though it seemed to be emotionally painful for him, being there by my side helped him cope. It was all he had the power to do. Who am I to deny him that. (By my second surgery, I asked him to be there at pre-op and post-op).

I was also completely enveloped in the book "Memoirs of a Geisha" by Authur Golden. I don't normally read Fiction. My reading choice is usually self help, if I read at all. This book was so good, and so realistic, it literally transformed me from a California woman facing breast cancer surgery into a Japanese geisha living in the early 1900's. I highly recommend to anyone facing surgery of any kind, get hooked on a book before going in and it will carry you through the process through the power of distraction.

After putting on the hospital gown with 3 holes (putting my head in the middle one and my arms in the other two before realizing all 3 holes are for the arms) I hopped into bed and waited for the flurry of attention and questions I was about to endure. They put an IV into the back of my hand and taped it down. It's a good thing I wasn't signing using sign language to communicate with anyone or I would need to resort to one-handed signs (I wonder what Deaf people do). Between each visit for IV insertion, blood draw and questionnaires, I delved into Japan a few pages at a time. I received a visit from the Cancer Center nurse navigator who advises breast cancer patients about recovery, showing me exercises to do post-surgery and encouraging me to follow them daily. Compared to the hospital staff I met so far, she was so nice. Please be sure to take advantage of any "navigation" services offered by your cancer center to help you through all the complexities of this journey.

Next they called the gurney chauffer to wheel my bed up to the radiation department. There I met an Oncology intern (this is a teaching hospital) who obviously found herself quite a catch, as her engagement ring had the largest diamond I have ever seen. Good thing I had that as a distraction, because the procedure of injecting the radioactive blue dye for the Sentinel Node procedure was excruciatingly painful. Using ultra sound to guide the needle, the radioactive dye is injected in the tissue surrounding the tumor (all around, under and on top of it). With each wince of my face, she apologized, but there is no getting around the fact that this stuff hurts when it is injected. That was the most painful part of my surgery and recovery process to date. Fortunately, it only lasted about 10 minutes.

While jumping back into time, and Japan (reading my book), trying to forget what I just went through, another gurney chauffer wheeled me over to an x-ray machine on another floor. Everyone I talked to about the book I was reading (technicians, nurses, gurney chauffeurs) had either read the book themselves or were aware of how good the book is. They were right! What a great coping tool to escape the possible anxiety of that day.

Jan, the technologist who "marked me up" for the Sentinel Node light show was so cool. I keep forgetting that I am now part of the "middle age" generation and there are so many professionals out there now that are "young and hip." She made me laugh. That made my day. While laying as still as possible under the x-ray machine, I watched the monitor to see the lymph nodes in my chest and arm pit begin to light up as the radioactive dye was reaching them. The first areas to light up were above my breast along the collar bone. The nodes under my arm pit did not light up until last. Jan marked my skin with a blue marker with circles in each place that lit up. Later in surgery Papa Smurf would follow these guidelines to know where to cut to remove the "Sentinel Nodes." I was worried that he would be cutting on all 10 circles that were made, but evidently the primary area that carries cancer from the breast is under the arm, so they do not cut out the nodes that light up elsewhere.

After my visit with Jan, yet another gurney chauffer returned me to the pre-op room where I got lots of reading done, and had another visit by the nurse navigator from the Cancer Center. This time, she gave me this adorable little pillow shaped like a heart to use as a cushion after my surgery. I had yet to learn just how handy this tool would be as resting my arm against my body and wearing a seat belt were very hard to do after surgery. (Be sure to ask if your Cancer Center has a nurse navigator. This person is a wonderful resource for recovery.) When I saw the gurney chauffer coming my way, I knew it was time to roll again. (wish I could have earned frequent flier miles that day)

My next stop was the, what should I call it, the surgery prep room. (Please don't quote me on this stuff, it's been too long for me to remember what things were called, and I don't usually pay attention to that technical stuff anyway.) In the surgery prep room I was all alone. Since they were kind enough to squeeze me in for an evening surgery, I didn't have other surgery-mates (co-patients? Surgery-pals?) to shoot the breeze with while waiting. Besides, I had my book and was enjoying every minute. I met the anesthesiologist, learned the procedure and answered some more questions. Then they left me alone in the room with a man sitting on a stool near the window. Beyond him I could see all the doctors and nurses milling around. I swear, it looked like Smurfville! Each person wore a different type of hat or head cover, but all were wearing Smurf-blue scrubs. Evidently, they wear different hats so they can recognize each other when their faces are covered. After naming my surgeon Papa Smurf, this sight was just too funny.

I don't know about you, but I am working to change an old habit of pre-judging people. I looked at the man sitting on the stool and automatically assumed based on the simplicity of his tasks I observed that he was not a doctor. He was probably a technician of some kind who could bring me a warm blanket or alert doctors if something were to go wrong. We chatted awhile, and I deduced that he also considered himself an amateur psychologist, the way he talked about patients and their common pre-operation fears. Little did I know, I was chatting with a real Psychologist whose job it was to help patients with those pre-operation fears. Teach me a lesson! Why do I tend to evaluate someone to a lesser degree of talent when I could just as easily assume they are far more capable? Just think of the doors we would open for others if we simply changed our perception of their abilities.

They forgot to turn my sleepy juice on in my IV before wheeling me into the operating room. They had a huge stereo on and jazz music was playing while the doctors and nurses talked about sports, and kids and the like. When they noticed I was still awake, someone said "oops, we forgot to turn the crank." They turned the IV on, and the next thing I remember is getting into my father's car, laughing like I was high on a whole bottle of champagne (gotta love those Demerol highs!). I spent more time at the hospital before my surgery than afterwards. I was in the car on my ride back to Charlie's house a little more than 2 hours after my surgery finished. I don't remember anything until the next day.

7/9/02—Cathy Update #4
(1 Day After Surgery)

Post-Surgery Update

I am home after my breast reduction surgery at Club Med (Sutter General). Arrived home last night at 10:30 pm. I feel fine. Spunky as ever. I will give more details later as I have been instructed to not use my left arm for the next few days. Must keep typing to a minimum. Boy that Dragon Naturally Speaking voice navigation software would be really helpful right now.

My procedure went without a hitch. They took 5 lymph nodes. Don't know why yet. Have a follow up appointment on Thursday morning to get my drainage tube and syringe removed (looks like a hand grenade, glad I'm not going to any airport) and will ask for more info from Papa Smurf.

I thought I was turning into a Smurf when I got home as my urine was blue. Blue dye from the Sentinel Node procedure. I took off the bandages about an hour ago and, low and behold, I've still got most of my boob. What a wonderful discovery. It's even a bit firmer than before, but I don't recommend this to others as a form of fighting gravity as we age. Even if it is a bit smaller than the other, I can follow the advice I got from my friend Fug's dad last Thursday, "What the Lord hath forgotten, you can stuff with cotton."

Gotta go now as my care giver wants me to stop typing. Between my mom and Charlie, I couldn't be in better hands.

Love you all!! Your prayers worked! Thanks.

Lopsided Cathy

p.s. Thank you for the flowers, I have received 3 so far today.

7/12/02—Cathy Update #5
(4 Days Post-Surgery)

Two Steps Forward Then One Step Back

I knew things were going along too well. I figured it was the incredible strength of all my loved ones being channeled to me because no one could feel this good so soon after surgery. With the exception of the constipating side effect of the Vicodin I took right after surgery (I'm still full of shit) and the fact that the most painful part of my surgical procedure was the radioactive dye they injected in my tumor area before surgery, I was feeling good enough to spend 30 minutes on the exercise bike this morning. I was feeling swell, so swell that I had to rush to the doctor's office this afternoon to have my breast aspirated (have fluid removed from under my skin). I started to grow a third boob under my arm.

I thought that I may be one of the lucky women who get to experience lymphedema, not into my arm, but into my breast and area under my armpit stretching into my back. Since the drain was removed yesterday, I thought I was leaking fluid into the tissue area of my surgery, however the doctor couldn't get any fluid out with the needle aspirator today. This may be the result of the hot weather (112 degrees) or just the way my body is healing. First, Papa Smurf warned me, "this is going to hurt like the dickens," then he inserted the thick needle under my arm, knowing full well I did not have feeling in that area. I guess you can call me "Numb Pit" as one of the side effects of surgery in this area is loss of feeling (and no more perspiration under my arm, which will save me 50% on deodorant from now on). Don't worry, I haven't lost any feeling in my heart. I just hope this swelling goes down before I begin to resemble Dolly Parton on the left side and remain Cher on the right. (Ruthy you don't know how close to home you hit when I read your card today and you called me such a "swell" friend. Stop that!)

My biggest disappointment was realizing I should stay in Paradise for a few more days so I can be close to my surgeon, when all I want to do is go home to Tracy and be close to my son Paul. I haven't seen him since the day before surgery. I cried. This hurts more than the radioactive dye did.

All this on a day when I bought the most beautiful moonstone locket necklace. This is not the good health that this stone is supposed to bring (but when you think of it, swelling is not a major medical problem). A friend of mine loaned me a handsome moonstone necklace to wear to protect my health from the cancer, however I have to give it back eventually and wanted to replace it as soon as possible with one of my own. My mom, her friend Alice and I took a stroll through the gift shops of Paradise Village this morning and the first store we walked into and the first case I looked in contained this beautiful moonstone locket. Now, I am a woman of science, but I believe in metaphysical forces to the extent that they are not harmful and don't cost a fortune. (Not as a replacement for medical treatment, but as adjunctive therapy) I have a magnetic mattress pad and place healing magnets near my surgery area as often as possible to speed recovery. I had my aura read by a friend of mine and plan to have a two-hour reading soon (she gave me a coupon!). I'll accept healing of any kind, in that aspect I am non-denominational.

Now for the scientific stuff… I hoped to be able to announce that "Node News is Good News" but actually the news about my nodes is only, fairly good.

My tumor was removed with clear margins except for the area nearest my skin (that area of skin was removed in surgery). The radioactive dye and the blue dye procedure found 5 sentinel nodes (2 in one lymph node region and 3 in another) It appears that my nodes are also highly motivated (just like me) which is why I have 5 sentinel nodes and not just one or two. Only one of the nodes shows a micro-metastasis. (an extremely small spread of cancer from the tumor into the lymph node) The size of the metastasis is small enough to expect that there was not enough time for the cancer to spread to other parts of my body, OR that if it did spread, the other region of metastasis is incredibly small and will most likely be killed by the chemotherapy treatments. If there happen to be other metastasis in my remaining lymph nodes, those would be small enough that the radiation therapy and chemotherapy will most certainly kill those. But that is unlikely, since the sentinel nodes only show one node with miniscule growth. So, there you have it. This is the reason I wanted sentinel node biopsy surgery. Both the doctor and I are comfortable that we do not need to take any more nodes. If not for this procedure, they would have likely taken at least 10 nodes or more, and I could run the risk that I wouldn't be able to move my arm around as freely as I can today. So I can "Just Say NO" to more node surgery. Another interpretation of this finding is, "we found it just in the nick of time." Had the metastasis been larger, there would have been more time for the cancer to spread to other parts of my body and possibly develop into larger tumors elsewhere.

So this is how my next few weeks look, barring any unforeseen 'swell' events. I will stay in Paradise until Monday morning to ensure my proximity to the doctor for a few more days and enjoy the powerful air conditioning system in this house compared to the wimpy one in the Tracy home (it has been over 100 degrees all week). Paul is asking his two bosses for Sunday off so he can come up to see me and drive me home on Monday. Tuesday July 16, I plan to participate in the Cancer Walk at work in front of Health Services at 12:15. I may bow out if the weather is too hot. I also have an appointment in town with a scalp specialist to talk about how to treat my bald head during my chemo treatments. Wednesday morning my mom is driving me back to Sacramento for my follow up appointment with Papa Smurf. I also have an appointment with a Nutritionist at the Cancer Center to discuss vitamin and mineral supplements. (You have never seen me more compulsive than to see the chart and multiple pill boxes I have filled with just the right amount of health pills for optimum recovery and anti-oxidant power. *I later abandoned this regime during chemotherapy under advice from my oncologist.*) Thursday I go back home to Tracy for a few days to be with Paul. Sunday morning I go back to Paradise to celebrate Charlie's birthday. Monday July 22 I go back into the hospital for surgery to have a port-a-cath inserted into my chest. This port and catheter will be used to give me the chemotherapy treatments and to do the multiple blood draws that will be done over the next 3 months. It will save my right arm from harm. Due to lymph node removal, my left arm is not to be used for injections and I must take care to avoid getting an infection in my hand or arm. July 26 I have an appointment with my oncologist in Stockton to schedule my chemotherapy treatments for the following 3 months.

I am as determined as ever to beat this thing. I was watching my mom and her friend Alice at dinner the other night. They were playing and arguing back and forth like I argue with my best buds. I've never seen my mom behave quite like ME before. What a joy, especially when I realize that 16 years ago, she was facing what I face today. Her tumor was larger, she had a mastectomy, but her metastasis was the same as mine. I want to be in my 60's and playing at the table with my best buds just like she is today. And I will. If you know me, when I set my mind on something, just try to get in my way, and watch yourself cower in fear as I trample all over you. (Oh, gee, that was a bit harsh. Actually my nature is far more manipulative so most victims don't even know what hit them)

Love you all. Keep those positive vibes coming my way. (send anti-swell vibes) The cards, flowers and gifts of large amounts of cash are also greatly appreciated.

Until the next update…

Ciao,

Cathy

p.s. go tell it on the mountain…permission to share…etc.

7/18/02—Cathy Update #6
(10 Days Post-Surgery)

"Listen to Your Body"

So, what happens when your body betrays you? I feel so good since my operation, I have been somewhat active. (For those who know me, that would be about 1/5 my usual pace) Papa Smurf kept telling me to do what I can, stop when it gets uncomfortable. I hadn't felt uncomfortable until the point when I began retaining liquid and he tried to aspirate on Friday, only to give up when nothing came out. Of course, 9 hours after arriving home in Tracy for the first time in a week, I was on the phone again needing more attention from the doctor. The left breast (or as Daniel Day Lewis fans may call "My Left Tit") was so swollen I was changing character from Dolly Pardon to Carol Doda. (Right side still stuck on Cher) I was afraid I would burst at the incision site. My mom, (my living guardian angel destined for sainthood) drove from Fremont (52 miles away) to pick me up in Tracy and drove me back to Paradise (over 80 miles) late Monday evening so we would be close by for my 8:30 a.m. appointment with Papa Smurf for a second attempt to aspirate. This time was successful (suck-cess-full) as 8 oz. was drained during this deflating experience and I am now more even. I guess you could say, it's like Cher-and-Cher alike (Sorry for the puns, I was twisted enough already without the cabin fever).

Now I am more balanced, I have decided to allow the brain to make decisions the body seems to be unaware are needed. I have a new routine, 4-up/2-down. I am now laying down twice each day for two hours to ensure I am getting enough horizontal time to allow the fluids in my body to do something different. I am also wearing a very tight bra to ensure that there is no room for more swelling and to keep my incision site from developing a thick scar from the tissue pulling constantly from extra pressure. (my friends are not the only support I get these days) At this point I am maintaining a moderate size and should make it until my second surgery on Monday July 22 where I can be aspirated again. (talk about ex-aspirating!…sorry) *I have no idea if my crude methods of lying down and wearing a bra helped. But even if it SEEMED to help, that in and of itself is help.*

This recent development has brought to my attention that during this phase in my life, I may plan things, but that doesn't mean I will get to do them. I firmly believe that flexibility is the key to success and so it must also be the key to accepting I don't have full control over my body at this time. It's times like this that we should be grateful… satisfied that we have selected enough good reading material to get us through these unexpected periods of forced rest. I just finished reading "Memoirs of a Geisha" and am now reading "It's not About the Bike" by Lance Armstrong. I haven't read a book for pleasure in so many years, this is such a treat. Until I get this meditation thing down, I consider reading fiction and biographies the same as meditation-lite. You can escape your own reality for awhile and live in someone else's story. Just remember to pick a book that makes you feel good. After experiencing the life of a Japanese girl sold into slavery, the more I read, the more grateful I became for my own life.

Today I had a consultation with Mike from the Salon and Scalp Clinic in town. What a gem! He spent so much time explaining to me what to expect from the chemo treatments and how to care for my scalp and skin, and then he wouldn't accept any payment. He also gave me some samples of a special shampoo and scalp treatment for chemo patients, Nioxin. (and you guys that are light on top, this shampoo and treatment will help stimulate hair growth!!!, no club membership needed) He was kind and caring and thorough. He informed me that there is a 99.99% chance of me losing my hair when taking AC chemotherapy. He also said one of the hardest things about cancer these days is losing your hair (because treatments are so much better than before). Think about how visual our society is. The top of the head and face (and many times more) are exposed everywhere we go. (I guess there is only ONE good use for a Burkah, now that I think about it) I will not only lose the hair on my head and body, but very possibly my eye brows and eye lashes too. He is having a "Look Good, Feel Better" workshop (sponsored by the local American Cancer Society chapter) for cancer patients in his clinic on August 19. By then, I should be bald as a cucumber. (Who invented that phrase?) We will learn how to apply makeup to draw in eyebrows and take attention away from our hairless features. Kind of a Tammy Faye support group (*This is a reference to her fame related to her heavy make up use. This was written years before she was diagnosed with her own cancer*).

My son Paul drove me to and from the appointment with Mark and sat in during the consultation. I cried on the way home, and he held my hand firmly, showing me the best way he could how much he cares. (He is suppressing a lot of his feelings about this so I wanted him to participate in the "hair experience" to give him a chance to express what he is holding in. Although he did not share his feelings, it must be tough to be a young man of 17, only child to a single parent, carrying the weight of Mom's cancer on your shoulders, in silence). I decided I wanted to cut my hair before starting chemo so I will be feeling better when faced with the emotional trauma of losing it all. I wanted the cutting of my hair to be a private and special ritual with Paul, and so it was. The braid lay in his room, about 15 inches long. He developed a sharp cramp in his wrist while cutting through it. (It may be gray, but it's thick) I am now sporting a short haircut for the first time in my life, compliments of Kathy, Paul's co-worker at Super Cuts (Another freebie). Spending today with him and overcoming my depression (at least for now) about my hair has moved me forward another step (I'll get into more details later about hair, since I have had long hair my entire life, this is a very sensitive subject for me which will no doubt need an entire update all to itself).

Medical update: Time to get technical. During my draining experience with Papa Smurf on Wednesday morning, I received more good news about my tumor evaluation. We already know that the margins were clear and that only one lymph node had micro-metastasis. Tests done during my needle core biopsy noted that the tumor was slow growing. Another test (Her-2 neu) done last week also confirmed that the type of cancer I have (had) is not aggressive. The hormone receptive status of the tumor is estrogen receptive positive and slightly progesterone receptive positive, another indicator that it is a slower growing type of cancer (*In retrospect, I don't think this is true, however it is an easier cancer to treat than estrogen receptor negative tumors*). The best news about the hormone receptive status is it means I have one more type of treatment I can take to double ensure I won't get this back. My cancer needs estrogen to grow. Tamoxifen (not fen-fen) is a hormone blocking therapy that I can take in pill form for 5 years to prevent any cancerous cells from absorbing estrogen. The chemotherapy will also cause me to go through menopause (fry my ovaries) so that I won't be producing much estrogen when this is all over. *Ha! I had no periods for 10 months, then they came back for 5 months, then they disappeared again for 4 months. Now, 5 years later, they are still with me. My hopes to never have periods again didn't come true.*

It Ain't Comin' Back!!

So, my next plan is for my second surgery on July 22 in Sacramento (Charlie's taxi this time) to have an access port inserted into my chest so that my chemo treatments can be dispensed directly into a main vein near my heart. This will prevent my arm veins from being damaged during my chemo and all my numerous blood draws can also be taken through this port. It will be a direct pathway to my heart. (sounds romantic) Papa Smurf was kind enough to offer to insert the tube about 1 inch below my right breast instead of the traditional location above the breast. This will allow me to continue to wear all those low cut, cleavage exposing dresses I own without any scars showing. (since the Dolly and Cher experience, I now have cleavage for the second time in my life. First time was during breast feeding). It ain't all it's cracked up to be (sorry, there I go again).

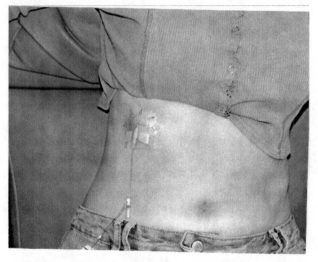

Most patients have a port inserted near their collar bone. Mine was placed over my lower rib cage for a less noticeable scar.

Then, July 26 I meet with my oncologist to discuss chemotherapy treatments, doses and scheduling.

Thank you again for the cards that keep trickling in. Thank you David for the flowers (and Lucy and Joanne and Leslie and Honey and the VEC) That check for $1000 from an anonymous donor was especially sweet. (psych!)

Until we read again,

cMc

p.s. Disclaimer about sharing info, same song, fourth verse....

7/23/02—Cathy Update #7
(15 Days Post-Surgery)

It's Not About the Breast

"It's Not About the Breast," She Says to Tour De Lance, "It's....
About....the....Haaaaaaair!"

Gimme a Head with hair

Long beautiful hair

Shining, gleaming, streaming flaxen waxen

(Sing Along: Lyrics by James Rado and Germoe Ragni from the Musical "Hair")

I'm a child of the 60's. Long hair has always meant a lot to me. When my mother cut her long hair in 1970 in favor of a Mrs. Brady pixie, I wouldn't speak to her. She bought a wig for me to brush and style because I no longer had her hair to play with. I have only truly cut my hair twice in my life (trims don't count). The first time was when I turned 30 and was going through my divorce. Change was needed. My hair was down to my knees back then. I had recently visited Washington DC and somewhere I have a picture of me standing in an alcove at the National Museum of Art at the Smithsonian, posing with my hair flowing behind me. My hair was a work of art (pre-gray, obviously). Several years ago I jumped out of an airplane (intentionally) and I have a video of my hair, flowing in slow motion in the wind as I prepared to jump (Silent Lucidity by Queensryche playing in the background). My name sign in sign language is "long braid." In the Deaf community, people are not known by the spelling of their name, but by name signs that are given to them, most often based on some physical attribute. I was known in the Deaf community as the interpreter with the long hair (most often worn in a braid). In the belly dance community (yes Virginia, the girl does belly dance) I have always thought that the dancers with long hair look truly authentic. Anything other than traditional seemed to me to be too American. Somehow I felt more confident because I had long hair. Perhaps they won't notice I don't have much skill if I look the part. I am truly an amateur dancer.

The second time in my life that I cut my hair was 6 days ago. Once again, change is upon me. I originally planned to wait until my hair started to fall out before cutting it. Hanging on desperately until the last possible moment to cling to this dead protein I considered such a large part of my identity. (Even though I know it is shallow to believe this way, I was surprised at how overwhelming the loss of hair is within our society. I didn't realize the impact, until it happened to me.) I was so depressed after visiting Mark at the hair salon and hearing how definite it was that I was going to lose my hair. My sister-in-law asked if I was going to cut my hair before it falls out so I could have some fun with different styles. I hadn't thought of that before. Then came the realization that cutting my hair now, before I begin chemo treatments, would be smart. I may better handle the emotional trauma while I feel well instead of when I am whacked on chemo. So, my son Paul cut my braid off and he is keeping it for awhile. (We will eventually donate it to the Cancer Society to make several natural hair wigs for children cancer patients) Paul happens to work for a popular low-cost hair salon chain, so after the braid came off, he took me to work with him and I received my first hair style ever. Tomorrow I have another appointment, with a "real" hair stylist, for a shorter cut and new color, something auburn (possibly puce). I may even get another cut and style before it falls out. Maybe even another color.

So, how do I feel about this short hair?

FABULOUS!!!! What the hell was I thinkin' all these years holding on to that funky old, split ends hair?

I love having short hair. What versatility! It's cool. I feel (and some say I look) younger. What a freeing experience. It's like discovering nudity. Those naturalists have something there (or should I say, nothing there). I can finally forgive my mom for cutting her hair (22 years is too long to hold a hair grudge).

Now I realize that losing my hair is not the most devastating part of my cancer experience. So far, my two surgeries haven't been so bad either. (yesterday's surgery went well, but I am still in pain, so pass me some more Vicodin honey) I still have to face the chemo and radiation treatments. I've only just begun my journey. Six weeks down, 20 weeks to go.

I see my short hair as a symbol of the new life I am facing ahead of me. So much soul searching going on inside my head these days. I am changing already, and I haven't even been through the worst of this yet. Tony Robbins would suggest that I anchor new feelings to this short hair and move toward new behaviors and beliefs. I am certainly appreciating my loved ones much more than before. Now, when someone asks me when the wedding is, I answer "next year" instead of "when the tax laws change." Somehow saving money doesn't seem as important as getting married. I have gained an incredible sense of appreciation for Charlie. He has been so wonderful through all of this. We have been planning the remodel on his Paradise home for at least a year now, so wouldn't it make sense for us to get married when I move up here next year when the remodel is complete? (*Hah! Anyone who has done a remodel knows that by the time this book gets published, the remodel isn't finished yet!*) I never thought I would think about doing something as old fashioned as getting married before I live with the man. Go figure.

Surgery update: Papa Smurf evened out Dolly again during my surgery yesterday. I have another appointment with him next week Tuesday to follow up on my surgery and even out Dolly again. (She is still swell, but less and less so as time goes on) The port and catheter insertion surgery went well, but I am still quite sore. The entire catheter is under my skin. There is a lump (hey, didn't I get that removed?) under my skin about two inches below my right breast. It is between my rib cage and my skin about the size of a quarter and 1/2 inch thick. The catheter membrane is right under the skin surface and that is where the IV for the chemo treatments will be inserted. The rest of the tube that leads to the vein in my heart is completely hidden, so I don't know where the heck it is under there. The reason he placed the catheter in my lower chest as opposed to my upper chest (the usual place) is to avoid scaring where it would be most visible (except during bikini season).

This Friday I meet with my oncologist in Stockton to learn about my chemotherapy treatment plan. The update after that appointment will probably be quite technical, so have your medical dictionary ready.

Until the next update…

Love you!!!

cMc

p.s. yes Virginia, you can share this info with your friends.

7/27/02—Cathy Update #8
(19 Days Post-Surgery)

It's Not About the Hair

And Tour de Lance responds to the naïve cancer patient, "It's not about the hair… it's about winning…no matter how long the race!"

I sit here on the eve before Lance Armstrong wins his next Tour de France race, contemplating my emotions from yesterday and reveling in my newly found strength. I am constantly amazed at the knowledge that is placed in front of me every day of this experience, as if I am being tested to see whether or not I will discover it and take advantage of what I see. I highly recommend to everyone who reads my updates to please take the time to learn how to shut the world off around you and listen to what's inside. If we quiet the mind long enough, things are revealed to us that wouldn't otherwise be obvious. (Contrary to what Timothy Leary would say, this can be achieved without organic or other mind expanding elements) I've never slowed down before. I didn't know what I was missing.

Not bad considering I haven't even opened the Meditation for Dummies book yet.

Yesterday was a hard day. I met with my oncologist Dr. Bangladesh to discuss my chemotherapy regime. After all was said and done I must admit I admire him and have faith in his knowledge and expertise. He has been very responsive to my requests.

As a recent college graduate (excuse me "returning student" as they called us old timers) and an employee of a research and development laboratory, I walked into his office with a list of questions that would cause most doctors to cringe. I did as much research as possible on line to discover what I could about chemotherapy options. I had the impression that my form of cancer was slow growing enough to warrant a regime of chemo-lite. I challenged his initial recommendation of AC (Adriamycin and Cytoxan) and was hoping to convince him that I could achieve the needed results by taking CMF (Cytoxan, methotrexate and 5-fluorouracil). My mother had CMF and didn't lose much hair (there I go again about the damn hair) and what is good enough for Mom is good enough for me. I was expecting the CMF regime would be less harsh than the AC. (These are the times when we learn just how little we know and how we allow ourselves to go down a path based on ignorance and hope). I lost sight of the fact that Mom's cancer was 16 years ago. New medicines are better than before. I also forgot about the fact I read over one month ago "those whose breast cancer comes back as a metastasis, don't often survive." My doctor only wants to fight back as hard as possible to prevent reoccurrence. I was also unaware that my tumor was not the 1.2 cm measurement I learned about from the ultra sound. The pathology report from my surgery measured it to be 2.3 cm at it's longest point (since it was shaped somewhat like squished silly putty).

His recommendation now, with the larger tumor size and metastasis in one lymph node, is to follow my 4 cycles of AC with 4 more cycles of Taxotere. There was a study released just this past May that shows promising results with this combination. (If you know of the study, please send it my way. Not that I don't trust, I just want to know more). This is good news and bad. I am lucky to be able to receive the benefits of new research, but will be on chemotherapy twice as long. After crying on mom's shoulder and challenging the doctor so I would better understand, he offered me the opportunity to get a second opinion and he offered to bring my case up to the monthly board of oncologists for discussion. Since the AC treatments will begin on August 8 and end October 10, there is time for me to learn and become more comfortable with this treatment decision before the Taxotere begins.

I spent the afternoon crying and surrounding myself with all the nourishing cards and gifts from all of you. I hung my cards up on my bathroom mirror and by ribbons on the wall while listening to "massage" music. Aromatherapy candles filled the room with soft fragrance while I hugged my huge teddy bear (thanks Jan) and soaked up all the love. (I received an e-mail from someone this morning that I hope to share with you later. It made a huge difference in how I feel today).

"Each friend represents a world in us, a world possibly not born until they arrive, and it is only by this meeting that a new world is born." - Anais Nin (thanks CC)

Do I want to be "comfortable" or do I want to survive? If Lance can handle Platinum treatments 5 days in a row, I can certainly handle AC + Taxotere (light weight compared to what he went through. My treatment only lasts 4 hours per cycle and is far less toxic). The timing of Lance Armstrong's Tour de France and reading his book while I go through this experience is one of those events I mentioned being "placed" in front of me. I find myself reading the Sports section of the newspaper for the first time in my life looking for a Lance update. I am not competitive by nature, but I guess it's time for me to step up to the plate. My Tour de Lance begins August 8, 2002 and ends near the end of February 2003 . (8 cycles of chemo followed by 6 weeks of radiation) "…it's about winning…no matter how long the race."

In his book I am learning how Lance went from being selfish to becoming selfless. I find this disease having a somewhat opposite effect on me. I am learning to be selfish for the first time. I have always spent time meeting with my many friends and giving people my time, such a precious commodity. The nature of my job is to serve people and give them my time and energy. After graduating from University of the Pacific in 2000 (6 years of part-time college during full-time work as a single mom) I found myself with time enough for a hobby, for the first time in my life. Now, I have a lot of time…to think. I apologize for not spending any time with my friends right now but the solitude is a sort of selfish sanctuary. I cherish it. It is helping me to cope. I may not go back to being the social butterfly I once was. I want more time with my son, he graduates high school 4 months after my treatment ends. I want more time with Charlie…wedding in October 2003? I want more time with ME.

The beauty of this e-mail thing is I have the chance to talk to all of you, at once. The efficiency freak in me loves that. I still feel like I am visiting with my many friends. I can read your e-mail replies and respond without having to drive out of town (which everyone lives outa town in California). This is my chance to still be with you, even though you are not here for me, you are THERE for me. This too helps me cope.

Sorry this update was not as fun as previous. I have been told I am having too much fun with my cancer. But today I'm kinda in a funk. Does that mean I am funky? Who invents these words anyway? Get George Carlin in here!

Luv ya!!

cMc

p.s. You know the routine, like shampoo…she tells two friends, then they tell two friends, and so on, and so on…. (gotta be over 35 to remember that commercial).

7/31/02—Update #9
(23 Days Post-Surgery)

Cathy Shares Reply

I received the message below from an acquaintance at work. I read it on the day after my "funk" day. After crying, I felt a new sense of hope. To have such support from someone who I only know casually at work brought me a new sense of belief in the awesome power of the human spirit.

Many others have sent me similar words of support, people I don't even know. Thank you!!!

Enjoy!!!

I just wanted to let you know I've been reading your updates with great interest and empathy. I believe writing to be an enormously effective outlet for emotion. When I experience a major life event, or even a significant ah-hah moment, words get so bottled up inside me that I can't rest or concentrate until I've written them all down. Feelings course out of my addled brain through whatever medium is at my disposal, clearing space for a small bit of sanity to return and give me some temporary peace.

I was leaving on a two-week vacation to Italy/Sicily with my daughter and mother on Saturday, July 6th. I stopped by the office Friday evening to tidy my desktop, having taken the day off to do some last-minute make-sure-you-have-enough-clean-underwear chores. Being the obsessive computer geek that I am (tee-hee!), I decided to check email one final time before leaving. I opened "Cathy Update 6/22," which had been forwarded from Tim that morning. This was the first I'd heard of your cancer, and I couldn't believe it. I double-checked the name on the email a couple of times and did all the stupid stuff people do when they've just heard awful news. (I had to check four different channels on 9-11 before I believed that happened, too.) Unfortunately, I couldn't dwell too much on your situation since I had a plane to catch in the morning. But I had a plan.

With the nine-hour time difference, flight delays, and various airport security/customs checkpoints, we flew into Roma late Sunday morning. The main goal of our vacation was to visit Sicilia and meet up with some family. However, the primary purpose of staying in Roma for five days (other than eating like pigs) was to attempt to see the Pope—something my mother's always dreamed of. I'd tried to arrange things state-side, without luck. He normally gives blessings on Sundays and audiences on Wednesdays, but that was all I could find out.

After arriving at the hotel and settling in, I mangled the native tongue in a lame attempt to communicate our request to the concierge (with both hands flailing, of course!). Eventually the poor guy scribbled down a phone number for me to call. I called it from the room, and the voice on the other end told me to be at such-and-such place Wednesday at such-and-such time and a van would pick us up. I figured we'd either end up in front of Papa or in a back alley with chalk outlines. But we appeared as instructed, and, after crossing some palms with the appropriate number of Euros, we were whisked away for the hour+ drive to Castel Gandolfo at typical Italian break-neck speed through some absolutely breathtaking rural Roman countryside.

"Papa," as the Italians refer to their Pope, had just been moved to his summer residence at Castel Gandolfo two days before we arrived in Rome due to his failing health. I discovered through our guide that things had been arranged for him to hold his Wednesday audience at Piazza del S. Pietro (the large plaza outside St. Peter's Basilica), but with the change in location he was now expected to "give the Mass" at his summer residence. This seemed to be a stroke of luck on our part, as I understood that many pilgrims hadn't been made aware of this.

When we arrived, the van took off (kind of scary, but what the heck I knew how to holler "taxi" in Italian) and we made the trek up the hill to a small piazza in front of the house. The Castel Gandolfo house was a much smaller and more intimate setting than St. Peter's, and was surrounded by the required number of tacky souvenir stands (dare I ask for Pope-on-a-Rope?) and various trattorias selling panini (sandwiches), dolci (sweets), and gelati (world's greatest ice cream!). I entered a small souvenir shop selling religious icons and purchased a few small items, including one small silver cross for E 0,88 (a little less than $1.00 US). I put the little bag in my purse and joined my family, who had bought gelato cones without me. But since we were near the Pope, I forgave them. :)

I knew we'd hit pay dirt when I noticed an inconspicuous wooden blockade at the house's courtyard entrance, by which stood a couple of guards wearing distinctive Vatican uniforms. They seemed to be quietly clearing people into the courtyard area, so I grabbed Mom and Amanda by the hands and ever so politely ("mi scusi," "permizzione," "grazie") pushed and shoved our way into the queue that had formed. We got the standard feel-up/feel-down security routine, and scooted past the swelling crowd. We were in! Mom still can't get over how I managed to pull that one off (me neither).

The courtyard was deceptively full but cozy, with typical old-world charm. There was a small patio in front of some French doors with steps leading up to the house. I looked above the doors and saw a terrace with a plate of what I sadly recognized to be bullet-proof glass behind a wrought-iron railing. Even with all the security measures at the airports and those I face at work each day, this was a sobering reality. I glanced around uneasily—who knew what was really on the agenda of all these strangers?

After about a half-hour of standing and craning our necks, the French doors opened. Cardinal Blah-Blah-Blah (first runner-up?) came out and announced the beginning of the audience. We all looked up towards the terrace as he told us what was on today's agenda; that Sua Santità (His Holiness) would discuss the Book of Daniel, and would welcome the groups from all over the world who had made special appointments. As he spoke, some more runners-up carried an ornate chair onto the patio and then, escorted by more Cardinals, Papa appeared and sat down.

Despite his physical deterioration, his voice rang out clear and loud. (The loud part was thanks to an impressive Papal sound system.) The groups were announced one by one, and he addressed them in their native tongue (he speaks eight languages). As he blessed the newly-married couples and reached out to touch the children, I glanced up at the terrace again and gulped with the realization that, over 20 years earlier, this frail man had almost lost his life in an assassination attempt. He could have easily appeared to us from behind the protection of that thick, greenish glass, but instead chose to remain approachable to the people. I was immediately humbled by his unfailing belief in the human element; my heart swelled with love and respect. No wonder the Italians love their Papa!

I thought of how we as Americans are taught from childhood to ignore and even shun people we don't know. "Don't talk to strangers," we tell our kids. "Don't take rides from strangers."

"Stay away from strangers." It's no wonder we're in a state of stressed-out paranoia all the time! It had almost cost the Pope his life—still, wasn't it better to approach people with an open heart than to walk around diverting glances? When she found out she had cancer, Erma Bombeck wrote about all the things she wish she'd spent more time on in her life. I barely know my next-door neighbors. I have no idea what my postman's name is, and he's delivered my mail for the last eight years. I don't want to leave this planet knowing that I could have made someone's day a little more pleasant just by calling them by name! I was truly ashamed of myself, and vowed to spend more time smiling at strangers and talking to the people in my small corner of the world.

When it came time for the blessing, I reached in my purse and got out the small bag of relics I had bought earlier. I dumped them into my hand and held them up high—three generations of my family together in Italy. We bowed our heads and received Papa's blessing.

I bought the silver cross for you.

———————

God Bless you Joan!

Pay it forward!

cMc

8/4/02—Cathy Update #10
(26 Days Post-Surgery)

Hello Dolly, well hello Dolly
It's so nice to have you back where you belong (not)
You're looking SWELL Dolly, I can tell Dolly
You've been showin', you've been GROWIN', you've been goin' strong
(Sing Along: Lyrics by Jerry Herman)

As you can tell by the song above, my week began with Dolly acting up again. I am happy to report by the time I am sending this message, Dolly is back to Cher-size again, and it looks like this problem is not coming back again. (regardless of what the lyrics say, I won't be singing "Dolly will never go away again!")

My cancer experience is becoming a series of Broadway musicals. Hair, Hello Dolly and Le Miserables, to name a few. As long as the characters in my story don't become those of horror movies the likes of Freddy Kruger or Jason, I'll be fine.

Thank you to my friends who replied to my "funky" message last week with words of encouragement, supportive blessings and a dictionary definition of the word FUNKY, no less. I also received encouraging information about my proposed chemo treatment, which support my oncologist's recommendation. Thank you to my bosom buddies (other Breast Cancer survivors) for continuing to be my e-mail support group.

Yet another jam packed week of experiences. I'll try to be brief (ha!). Typing is also becoming a chore since I am letting my fingernails grow out (a luxury sign language interpreters never have) and they are totally getting in the way and hitting the wrong keys (but they look fabulous). Yet the spell check won't allow imperfection so you'll never know the difference.

Last week included some more "normal" activities for me as I am getting back into the swing of my old existence. I had a belly dance weekend last week (observing, not participating). The local dance troupe performed at Starbucks Saturday night and the following day I drove to Oakland for a dance festival where I had the opportunity to see my instructor (Nanna) and her troupe perform. She is incredibly graceful, and she was wearing.... A WIG! I now notice that many dancers wear long hair wigs when they perform, to have that "authentic" look I was talking about earlier. Ha! I didn't need that long hair after all. (By the way, just love my short hair, love it, love it, love it) At the festival I bought two more scarves to cover my head when the hair disappears. Fortunately I am experienced at wrapping turbans, thanks to my dance costume experience, and I am actually looking forward to creating some pretty head wraps with my new fabrics. If I don't feel like wearing my wig, I can also pretend I am a Muslim woman and wear scarves in their fashion. The options are limitless.

I don't know if watching dancing is as tiring as doing it, but I did notice a lot of pain in my porta-cath area that weekend. Once again I find myself doing too much. Since I paid so much attention to this pain, I decided to name my port and catheter "Cathy-ter." Makes it easier to reference later on, besides, the other two bumps on my chest have names (Dolly and Cher), might as well give my third boob an identity too. Charlie calls it "Alien" since it is located near my stomach and bulges out of my lower rib as if it is about to jump out and stick to his face. (Had to see the movie to understand that one) Fortunately, as of today, Cathy-ter is feeling much better. I barely notice her now that my skin has grown to allow for the bulge and she is hidden behind Cher from my eye's view.

Sunday was also the day Lance Armstrong won the Tour de France, again. I tried to finish reading his book before he crossed the finish line, but I forgot about the 9 hour time difference between here and France. He beat me. That evening on my way back from Oakland, I stopped for my monthly full-body massage by Joe (I needed to be kneaded). Since Dolly was feeling swell, we actually taped her up so she had support while I lay on my back. I got a "pregnancy" massage since I can't lay on my stomach. It not only felt wonderful, it was extremely therapeutic. 24 hours after my massage, Dolly began to deflate (the Hindenburg is going down!) for the first time since my surgery 3 weeks ago. I believe the massage stimulated my lymph system and kicked it back into gear to reabsorb the liquids that were causing my swelling. (Theory only, no proof)

I have been struggling to research information about antioxidants and chemotherapy. There isn't anything out there. Since my diagnosis, I started taking mega-vitamins to help me stay as healthy as possible. All the doctors I have talked to say there is no proof that anything other than a daily multivitamin does any better for our health. I wanted to take antioxidants and extra vitamins (especially vitamin C (to fight colds) and vitamin E (to fight blood clots in Cathy-ter)) during my chemotherapy treatments, but my oncologist discouraged me in regard to the antioxidants. His philosophy, which makes sense, is that antioxidants will fight against the chemotherapy. The point of chemo is to kill cells (preferably cancer cells, but unfortunately other fast growing cells die too). The purpose of antioxidants is to prevent cells from dying, therefore, it may actually prevent the chemotherapy from doing it's job thoroughly. So, I finally got an answer to my mega-vitamin question Monday night....I got sick. I came down with a cold, nothing unusual (sore throat, chest congestion followed by sinus congestion days later) but a cold none-the-less. I'm not even on chemo yet, and I got sick, while I was taking mega-vitamins. So, this is one of those "signs" that I am interpreting to mean "don't waste your money on the 'mega', go back to 'multi' and your odds of avoiding illness are the same."

I may have caught the germs from a visit to my primary care physician that day (doctor's offices are FULL of germs). It was a wake up call of how easy it will be for me to get sick when my immune system is defenseless during chemo. I'm thinking about becoming a cross between Howard Hughes and Michael Jackson and wearing a mask on my face and washing my hands 20 times a day. (Yet another use for a Burkah?) I have figured out a few ways to cut down on sharing germs. I now use my own pen when signing credit card receipts and other "outside" paperwork and I use a paper towel or tissue when touching anything in a public restroom. (yuck eeew)

Tuesday I had a follow up with Papa Smurf to further deflate Dolly. On the drive up to Sacramento (via Mom's taxi service, if not for my cold, I would have driven myself) we stopped in Stockton to pick up a compression sleeve for my left arm. I am not currently showing any signs of lymphedema (swelling) in my arm, but I don't want to take any chances of ever developing it. I hear, once it starts, it is very difficult to get back down to normal. So whenever I exercise my arms rigorously or whenever I fly in a plane (pressurized cabin) I will be wearing this tight sleeve to prevent any excess fluids from filling into my arm. *Lymphedema is a condition where fluids build up in the arm because the lymphatic system is not functioning to carry toxins and fluids out of the body through the lymph nodes under the arm.*

While in Sacramento I attended a few events of the California Youth Leadership Forum for Disabled High School Students (YLF). For the past 11 years I have volunteered (with my employer's support) at this event by being an interpreter or a counselor and also coordinating their talent show. It was hard not to be involved this year because it is such an incredible experience, but I was fortunate that my cold didn't keep me down too much and I was able to attend the talent show (Tues. night), mentor's luncheon (Wed. noon) and closing ceremonies (Thur. afternoon). [I will write more about this event in a future e-mail update. Too much to cover here but oh so worth hearing about, trust me.] One of the keynote speakers at the luncheon is a dear friend of mine, David Roche (davidroche.com). As he spoke about his disability (facial difference) as a gift, I also recognized that my cancer experience is also a gift. My perception of life has expanded since this ordeal in ways that never would have happened if not for going through this. David and I had a wonderful discussion that afternoon, it was for me something he would call "a moment of Grace." I hope that each of you are lucky enough to know someone who provides for you the opportunity to philosophize about life. If you don't know that someone, then why not BE that person for someone else. Either way the synergy that is created in these friendships benefits both parties.

Friday was a combination of test and medicine. The test, a CT scan of my torso (chest, abdomen and pelvis) and the medicine, the movie Austin Powers III. For the 10:00 CT scan, I had to drink a Barium shake one hour before my appointment and I couldn't eat or drink anything for two hours before or after. I was so tired from my cold, I didn't want to give up sleeping in during the morning. So, I woke up at 6:30, ate breakfast, and went back to bed at 7:00. I woke up again at 8:30, drank the Barium (that is not Bay Rum) and got ready for my appointment. It didn't taste as bad as I thought it would, another marvel of modern medicine. The scan also required an iodine injection via IV to be administered during the scan. The IV made me warm all over (felt like a shot of good single malt) and the test was done in a few minutes. (Can you tell I miss drinking alcohol?*) That afternoon my son Paul and I went to the movies. Reader's Digest says "laughter is the best medicine" so I took their advice. They were right.

* Cathy's heritage in a nutshell…I may come in a Portuguese package, but my wallet is Scottish and my liver is Irish!

This is getting long enough, so I better stop. Please let me know if you feel inundated by my updates and I'll be happy to unsubscribe you. This, if you can't already tell, is my therapy, but it is far cheaper than a shrink and it keeps me bonded to all of you who read it. Feeds the soul, you know.

I start chemo treatments on Thursday, August 8 so next week's update should be interesting, or maybe non-existent, depending on how I feel. Don't worry, I'll send something out eventually. You can't shut this girl up at this stage, this is becoming a habit.

Smackeroos,

cMc

p.s. spilling these beans is OK by me (in keeping with this week's Tracy Bean Festival theme)

7/28/02–8/1/02 California Youth Leadership Forum for Students with Disabilities

This section of the book was not an update. It is being added here to further explain and share with you the wonder of this event.

For decades there have been youth leadership events throughout the country for diverse populations of Hispanics, African-Americans, Asians and other cultural minorities. Their civil rights movement was in 1964 and since then many organizations and non-profits have been formed to help the youth of their culture develop a sense of identity, pride and leadership skills to make a difference in our nation's future. Not so for students with disabilities.

People with disabilities did not acquire their civil rights until the passage of the Americans with Disabilities Act in 1990, 26 years later. Because of Public Law 94142 in 1974, most students with disabilities are mainstreamed into local high schools and may never meet another person in their life who has the same disability they have. There are still schools for the Deaf and schools for the Blind because of their unique learning and language needs, so these two disability communities have strong cultural connections and sense of pride in their disability. Not so for other types of disabilities.

I am proud to have been a part of the California Governor's Committee on Employment of People with Disabilities when we developed the first Youth Leadership Forum for Students with Disabilities in 1991. Our forum is now duplicated in over 30 other states and there is also a National Youth Leadership Forum for Students with Disabilities in Washington D.C. This forum is an opportunity for students with disabilities to realize for the first time that they are part of a culture with a long history of political activism to bring about their civil rights, accessibility and accommodation to participate as citizens of this country. For many, it is the first time they are away from their parents (for some, an escape from overprotective environments). For some it is the first time they meet someone who has the same disability they have, and thus share the same experiences. For all it is an experience they never dreamed of…being a teenager and being accepted and respected by their peers.

It Is Pure Magic

I'll never forget the first year. There were two young men sharing a room with their attendant care giver. They both used powered wheelchairs to get around and neither had ever had a friend in a wheelchair before. They became fast buddies. At one point, they had wheelchair races down the hall with other students cheering them on from inside their dorm rooms (so not to get run over). We did not encourage such behavior, but how can you resist letting them enjoy each other. The life expectancy of one of them was just a few years more, and he did indeed eventually pass away before his 23rd birthday.

For YLF we transport 60 high school sophomores with disabilities from all over California via train, plane, para-transit (wheelchair accessible transportation), parents etc. to California State University Sacramento for 5 days that change their lives forever. We are emphatic in selecting diverse types of disabilities, ethnic backgrounds and geographic regions of the state so our forum is a true representation of our state's population. There are small group activities, each group consisting of 10 students with different disabilities, where the opportunity to share personal experiences and talk intimately empowers them. There are "student only" small group sessions where they can share personal discussions about dating, driving a modified vehicle or dealing with difficult parents. There are large group activities where guest speakers with disabilities share where they came from and how attitude makes all the difference in success. There is a technology and resource expo so students can learn what accommodations are available for them, and what organizations there are to help them through school and find employment. The students tour the state Capitol, meet with legislators and learn about the political process in which they have the opportunity to initiate change. The mentor's luncheon is an opportunity to meet professionals with similar disabilities to learn from, (and a chance to get away from the awful dorm food). There is a talent show, where no matter what talent you display will be received with a huge round of supportive applause. There is the dance, for many their first, where wheelchair users form snake lines (led by someone with an electric powered chair) and unique forms of dancing are the norm.

Five days of these activities, while living in the dorms, makes for life-long friendships. Discovering you are an integral part of a community you had no idea existed, is priceless. This forum is one of my favorite events. It feels good to volunteer and make a difference. The last day of the forum is quite emotional as fast friends leave each other hoping to never loose touch. The difference in these students faces, from the day they arrive compared to the day they leave, is tremendous. "I once was lost, but now I'm found. Was Blind but now I see." (except for the Blind students, who are still blind when they leave)

Students attend this forum at no charge. The forum us sponsored by donations to the Friends of the California Governor's Committee for the Employment of People with Disabilities, the Employment Development Department and the Department of Rehabilitation. For more information, please go to www.disabilityemployment.org.

8/11/02—Cathy Update #11
(33 Days Post-Surgery; 3 days after
1st AC Chemo Treatment)

AB FAB and Pill Stuff

I am doing my best to get this message to you in a timely manner. Now that I realize these updates are becoming more than "brief" and now people outside of my work place are wanting to receive them, I will soon be pursuing new avenues of sending out my e-mail updates to avoid using my work computer in the future. Although I believe these updates are a benefit to our current Cancer Awareness Campaign at work, I am sure the continued use of this avenue for my updates is inappropriate. So if you have tips or ideas of how to use DSL or cable modem systems at home please send your advice or cautions my way. You may soon be getting my updates from "Teenwolf" or "DonutDude" if I need to switch over to my son's e-mail account.

GOOD NEWS!!! I Feel AB FAB! (absolutely fabulous) With the exception of being Goombay (Gumby with a Caribbean twist), I have felt no nausea or unpleasant side effects from my chemotherapy treatment last Thursday. I do have the anti-nausea medication side effect of inability to write, type or think clearly, and stumbling is a bit of a problem too. (reminds me of a few good parties I've been to) But compared to what I have heard could happen, I'll take this simple state of stupor any day!

Where is my brain? I don't know if it is the actual chemotherapy itself or the three medications I was taking to combat these possible side effects that leave me quite incapacitated in the brain function area. I had a slight headache the first few days and was flush with a red face and chest. I had just a slight fever (2 degrees above normal). I am now down to just one pill, which prevents nausea but keeps me stupid. Other than these symptoms, I am ecstatic to be feeling so well right after my treatment. Just don't put me behind the wheel of a car or ask me to solve any problems that need a real answer. I can certainly begin to empathize with people who experience the side effects of brain injury. I search for ideas or try to find ways of expressing what is in my mind, but reading what I have written, I need to rewrite it all over again. And again.

These "mess-up-my-head" drugs are as follows: Pill A) Metoclopramide 10mg (generic for Reglan) two pills four times a day for two days. This is to be taken 30 minutes before a meal and it slows down the digestive system and sedates the esophagus to prevent any reflex reactions should I feel the urge to vomit (ew). This one also has a tendency to make me a bit restless, as I want to climb the walls and take a nap at the same time. Pill B) Dexamethasone 4mg (generic for Decadron) two tablets twice a day for two days. This is a corticosteroid that reduces swelling and inflammation to prevent allergic reactions. Last night I just finished taking the last dose of these two pills. In the twisted family tradition of pomp and circumstance, my mother brought them to me while wearing a tall blue Marge Simpson wig while I donned the wavy gravy wig for the pill taking ceremony. The only thing missing was crowns and scepters. Yes, we's all still wiggin' out at this house when it comes to celebrating my treatment.

I still have one more pill to take to prevent nausea, Lorazepam 5mg (generic for Ativan). It says it is for treating anxiety. I can take it every 6 to 8 hours or as needed. I don't expect to use it much longer as I am anxious (ha) to get these pills out of my system so I can get back the brain I so desperately need to continue functioning at what I consider my normal level.

I wanted to be sure to let you all know as soon as possible how well I am doing, however I will need to wait and mail you another update in the next few days with more information about the Chemotherapy process and my events of the past week. It seems the brain waves to the fingertips are not coordinated enough under these drugs to allow me to compose text well enough to explain myself. In a few days, when the drugs are done and my brain returns, you will get the old snappy Cathy back, ready or not.

Meanwhile, know that my first treatment was comforting and successful thanks to the prayers and grace you have all bestowed upon me. Thank you for keeping me in your thoughts. Many more updates will follow.

Love,

Goombay Cathy

Spread the word, and keep it simple so I can understand it when I read it again later.

8/13/02—Cathy Update #12
(2 Days Later)

First AC Treatment

Finally my head clears from the fog. Poor you, another long update to read. (Masochist!) Many people say my last update didn't seem unclear at all. If you only knew how many times I rewrote it and then had Charlie edit the final version. OK now, where did I leave off?

Tuesday August 6th (two days before my first chemo treatment) I had a Muga Scan. I went into the hospital fully expecting to have my face placed on a photo copy machine or read by a bar code laser. (not!) The MUlti Gated Acquisition test evaluates how strong my heart is to ensure it can withstand the chemo treatments. First they drew my blood and mixed it with radioactive dye. I returned a half hour later to have the mixture injected into my vein and my heart was scanned during several full beating cycles. One of the good things about going through this experience is I now know just how well my body is functioning. I have had so many tests. It's a shame we can't afford to have all these tests done when there is nothing wrong with us, just to keep the hypochondria away. Later that day I stopped into work to listen to a presentation about Peregrin, a molecular targeting radiation therapy procedure under research at UC Davis. I wanted to know if I could benefit from this study. I discovered that we are still too far away from clinical trials, and besides, this is really intended for end-stage cancer treatment. My radiation therapy will be more like a "clean up" procedure as opposed to a tumor shrinking treatment.

I set aside Tuesday afternoon for special preparation for my chemo treatment. A friend of mine from the local belly dance troupe came over and decorated Cathy-ter with a henna tattoo. Henna is used to decorate the hands and feet of women from Middle Eastern cultures in preparation for weddings and other special occasions. I wanted to celebrate my chemo treatment in the same way. (And I wanted to surprise the nurse when she went to insert the needle into my port). Many people may view going into a chemo treatment as a solemn experience. Oh contraire! I embrace the experience as a celebration of life. I am accepting this special fluid that is going to help save my life. What's not to celebrate? *Each week I decorated my Cathy-ter site with something new to make the RN smile while giving me chemo.*

Wednesday I headed back up to Smurf Land. I attended a free nutrition class for chemo patients offered by the Cancer Center. They offer the awesome free services of a nutritionist and nurse navigator. (I call the nutritionist Sue Hagen Das. If you knew her real name, you would understand why. No one is beyond special naming conventions in Cathy's Cancer Trip). She recommended several things I need to do to help the chemo process go more smoothly; drink a gallon of water every day to flush the system and keep me…"regular;" eat lots of protein to rebuild my red blood cells; eat small-portion meals several times a day to prevent any hunger-related queasiness and prevent over-stretching my stomach which can also lead to digestive discomfort. Other tips include avoiding odiferous foods and fatty substances. I stocked my refrigerator with lots of yogurt and quick simple meals. Fortunately I have been one of the lucky who have ZERO problems with eating so far. Keep your fingers crossed that this remains true for the rest of my treatments.

Wednesday was also a sad day for me when I realized that it was my last check up with Papa Smurf for 3 months. Have you ever been depressed that you aren't going to see your doctor? That's how much I love this guy. I gave him a copy of my updates, added him to my e-mail update list and snapped a photo with him and his way-cool nurse. (He loved the henna tattoo I prepared for my chemo treatment!) The good news is I will still see him every 3 months for the next year and then every 6 months for a few years after. Cool!

My son Paul works for a low price hair salon chain and gets a 40% discount on products. I asked him to buy me some large bottles of the Nioxin shampoo and scalp therapy before he quits his job next week so I can take advantage of his company perk. I was never so proud as when I came home Wednesday to find 2 one-gallon bottles of shampoo and conditioner sitting on the counter. (OK, first was shock, then was pride). After explaining to me that he couldn't pass up the opportunity to save over $100 and that this would last me a life time… he said Happy Birthday and Merry Christmas. (Gotta love 'm). So, please let me know if you are a bosom buddy and I will be happy to give you some Nioxin, free of charge (I'll bring some down when we visit Dennis!).

Thursday was THE DAY! I entered the Cancer Center ready to give "henna shock" to anyone willing to look. (My treating oncologist is on vacation, so he'll have to wait until the next tattoo for his treat.) I walked into the "Chemo lounge" with my bare mid-drift top and hip hugger blue jeans and said hello to the 4 elderly men sitting inside. One of them said, "your missing part of your shirt." I introduced myself and asked if there were any other Thursday regulars... John is it. He is in for fluids once each week, not even a chemo patient. One man hurried out to have a cigarette as soon as his treatment was done. (Damn you Phillip Morris)

The lounge is lovely. I sat in the lounge chair that overlooks a man-made lake with wall-to-wall windows on two sides. There are lots of large plants, my own TV set, videos, books, magazines, pillows, blankets, you name it...and the coolest nurse, Ses. When she saw the henna tattoo she cracked up and left the room to compose herself (success!). She brought back two nurses for show and tell. I also came equipped with a very special prop. My friend Pam sent me this little red paper cocktail umbrella to put on my "chemo cocktail." (The AC looks like a Cosmopolitan heavy on cranberry juice) When Ses left the room to mix my potions I told her "I like it shaken, not stirred!" Once my "juices were flowing" (tsk, tsk) we hung the umbrella from the IV bag so I could have my chemotherapy in style. I think we'll bring pineapple next time.

First I was given an IV with Decadron (anti-swelling) and Anzanet (anti-nausea) followed by a Saline flush. Ses informed me to make sure that during each procedure I check that it begins with a Saline flush of Cathy-ter and ends with 3cc of Heparin (anti-clotting agent). Then I was given Ativan (anti-anxiety/nausea). The Adriamycin was given to me in a "push" by alternating Saline with injections of the Adriamycin from a huge syringe over the course of 15 minutes. (looked like something out of the movie Clockwork Orange) I told Ses this makes her my "pusher." Then she hung the Cytoxan IV bag, which dripped for about an hour, followed by a Heparin flush. Total time of my treatment would be about two hours if not for her running around and treating other patients. I actually enjoyed the experience. The people are nice. I can snack and drink liquids while hooked up. I can walk to the bathroom (important feature) with my little IV pole on wheels. Both mom and Charlie were with me so I had lots of company. I only felt a little different when I left, mostly from the Ativan, which made me a bit groggy. The following few days at home were mostly that, groggy, with a little headache and flush face and chest. Not at all bad, not at all. I've had hangovers far worse than this. (I've had relationships far worse than this, and they lasted longer than 6 months.)

Friday I received flowers and the card read "for Dolly, Cher and Cathy-ter." I am happy to announce that Dolly is no longer with us, it's just Cher and Cher alike. No more musicals, as far as I can predict.

I find myself in the most unusual state of…lull. From the day of my diagnosis until my first chemo treatment my life has been a complete whirlwind. Doctor's appointments, consulting, tests, talking to other survivors, reading, researching, driving, preparing, praying, rejoicing, typing updates (therapy), and every now and then, a few tears. These past few days, at times I feel overcome with exhaustion (This is not a complaint. I'll take tired over nausea any day). Sometimes I have plenty of energy, then all of a sudden, wham, it's all I can do to get up and go to bed. I read, watch movies, make audio tapes, talk on the phone, sleep, eat, and pretty much do… nothing. What a change. I intentionally have nothing planned because I don't trust I'll be able to follow through with any commitments due to lack of energy. I have blood work on Thursday. That's all I have planned.

I am armed with an arsenal of reading for spiritual growth. I plan to use this time to recover my red blood cells and heal my soul. I've been given this gift of time and a second chance to develop a stronger spiritual self. This will help me heal physically too. Another reality about this "lull" time is there won't be much information to report in my updates. (Except when the hair falls out, that'll be newsworthy) Most of the "data" about my cancer experience has passed. Now, you poor souls, get to read future updates from the ramblings of a woman with nothing but time on her hands. Egad! These next few weeks I want to review details that I didn't have time to explain in my past updates so far; the procedures on the day of surgery, the Youth Leadership Forum experience, what I am learning from my readings, yadda, yadda, yadda. This will be like one of those movies where you'll turn to the person next to you and say, "is this a flashback?" Bear with me. As long as you are willing to stay tuned, you all get to be my group therapy session. (I never did follow through with my promise to write about my surgery day and YLF. I never ran out of subject matter while writing my updates. In this book I took the opportunity to follow through with that promise by inserting these stories between my updates.)

Bye for now,

the Princess of No-nausea

cMc

p.s. yack it up!

8/18/02—Cathy Update #13
(6 Weeks Post-Surgery, 10 Days After
1st AC Chemo Treatment)

"The Answer My Friend, Is Blowin' in the Wind,
the Answer Is Blowin' in the Wind."
(Sing Along: Lyrics by Bob Dylan)

I sit here on the patio swing as the morning sun rises. I'm in heaven, at home in Paradise. The bells from the Serbian church ring in the back ground to serenade the sounds of the squirrels scrambling from tree to tree and the magpies screeching from the tree-tops. Occasionally the wind chimes ring and the tree leaves rustle as the delta breeze blows through. We bought the chimes just before my surgery knowing their sound is healing to the soul, but for some reason they have never chimed before, even when the wind was up. The winds have changed, and so have I.

People think I am crazy when I talk about moving up here and commuting 2 hours one way to work. They just don't understand how much I love my job and how spiritual the space is that I will live in here. I believe two of the most important aspects to surviving in our modern society are to love what you do and to find a nurturing spiritual space to live in. I feel sad for those who have yet to discover these two aspects in their life. I haven't changed my path, for I have been blessed with a career choice and partner that fulfill my purpose on this planet. I still plan to move up here when my son graduates from high school and we continue with our remodeling plans for expanding the house and upgrading it's worn out infrastructure. What has changed is my approach, my perspective, and the depth of my appreciation for all that I have and for those who surround me.

Deep Stuff Huh!

Can you tell who has been reading spiritual growth books? Those of you who know me well are aware that I tend to WAY get into what I am focused on, sometimes at the expense of those around me who I have been known to bull doze over in my pursuit. (sorry!) Just this week I found myself mulling over henna tattoo web sites copying designs and contemplating my next tattoo design to make the chemo nurse smile. I drew for hours, developing a cramp in my wrist before realizing, "don't go overboard, it's just one day in the life." But I feel so good I can't stop myself from behaving impassioned about everything I do. Yesterday Charlie and I did vine-work in the back yard, separating the rose vines from the trumpet vines that grow together along the back garden fence. I climbed up the oak tree and cut down the jasmine vines that have grown up into the branches and Charlie and I worked together untangling the vines and spreading them along the fence to continue the curtain of jasmine that envelopes the patio. This is heaven. Physically connecting with nature is healing, but once again I remind myself to slow down and realize, "this is just one day in the life." When you live so focused on the "here-now" (Wayne Dyer's word) each day is so much richer.

Last night I was concerned that perhaps I did too much. I remember someone telling me that their carpel tunnel surgery was caused by "gardening" and I started worrying that I worked my left arm too hard and may develop lymphedema…and I left my compression sleeve at the Tracy house. For the first time since my surgery, I felt fear. Charlie, my angel-in-training, ran to the store and bought me an ace bandage to wrap my arm with. I unwrapped the Lymphedema book that I bought as a gift for a bosom buddy and I read how to wrap my arm. (thank you Donna for your gift of the Lymphedema book, that I also left in Tracy) The book said not to wrap my arm without training, I may do more damage than good. I wrapped up anyway, making sure the circulation was still good in my hand. I left it on for about an hour, all the time thinking, "is this right? It's Saturday night, who could I call to ask what to do?" Then I thought about what I have been learning this week in my readings and audio tapes. "I create my own reality." I remembered earlier this week when I ate some "left overs" (a real no-no for chemo patients because of possible bacteria concerns and weakness to fight them) and I started feeling queasy just thinking about what I had just done. Immediately I realized that it was my thoughts causing the feeling, not the food (it was only 10 minutes after I ate) and I stopped feeling queasy, instantly. I never got sick, because there was nothing wrong with the food, I just feared there was.

I remembered a quote from Brenda Premo (a phenomenal blind woman and the past director of Department of Rehabilitation in Calif.) that I often use in my disability awareness training. "FEAR is an acronym for False Evidence Appearing Real." If I can focus my energy on healing my arm from the possible damage I may have caused, instead of applying external pressure (bandage wrap that is possibly done wrong) and if I focus on my arm healing and not on it swelling, then perhaps I can influence what will happen to it. (wow, grammar check hates this sentence) So, I am not going to allow fear to take over. Today my arm feels fine, just a little tired. From now on, this experience has taught me to be more cautious with my arm, which in turn will prevent me from the fear that could have ruined such a beautiful day.

I know I was planning on using this time to write updates about previous experiences I haven't detailed to you yet, but I am inspired instead to share my NOW experience which is so wrapped up in spiritual growth. (seems that "wrap" is the theme for today. Perhaps I should write a 'rap' song about it. Not! Or would that be "knot!") Don't worry, I'm not coming over to your house on Saturday morning and handing you a pamphlet and I'm not going to e-preach at you, I just want to share with the you names and titles of what I am reading if you should choose to read them yourself.

It's all about energy. [As an aside, there is a blue jay taking a bath in the bird bath right now.] I believe a lot in this energy stuff as I have done my best to exclude myself from any experiences or people who may drain me of my energy while I am healing. I have been very secluded lately, the opposite of my usual gregarious, outgoing, ever expending-energy-on-others, self. I also used to scurry about at a hundred miles an hour, packing into my day as much as I possibly could fit. I am a Covey disciple with 14 years of Franklin organizers that document not just what I did, but who I talked to and their phone numbers. I used to think that the success in "highly effective people" meant cramming as much 'doing' in to the day as possible. I think I missed Covey's point. I think he meant to create a system that allows us to be more present in the task at hand because we are able to organize our time and not worry about other things while we are in the present. Yesterday, Charlie and I were sitting side-by-side in our little garden of Eden (doing Adam and Eve stuff, no, we were "being" Adam and Eve) and he said, "It's so nice to just "be" for awhile." I have spent too much time doing and not enough time "being." I have allowed our Euro-American culture to dictate how I live my life. I now choose to shift my behavior to a different cultural perspective, one that focuses energy on "being" and not just "doing." [A squirrel just ran down the palm tree being chased by some birds]

I walk slower, I take more time to sit…and think. (part of the reason I can do this is because of my disability leave from work. The challenge is to continue to do it when I return.) When I was getting my tires rotated the other day (the car's tires that is) I walked down to the coffee shop, had a bite to eat, read some more in my book by Wayne Dyer entitled "Your Sacred Self" and enjoyed the time. I used to stress about finding time to squeeze in those little time consuming chores like tire rotation, oil change, doctor's appointments, etc. Now, I can enjoy relaxing while waiting. Relaxing is something foreign to me, something I now choose to do more of. I look forward to working as part of our new Work-life Balance division (spawned by a recent reorganization) influencing our work place to allow people to alter their work schedules and let them spend more time in their life "being" while they are able to do these little chores that are so stressful to the 9 to 5 population.

I am also listening to the audio tapes "Anatomy of the Spirit" by Carolyn Myss. I have many others too (thanks to a loan from Ilene Goodwoman, and a good woman she is!) but this set is the largest. I knew I was meant to learn from Carolyn by several events that brought me to her. Charlie's cousin Sandy came to visit him the evening I had to rush back to Sacramento because Dolly was acting up. If not for Dolly, I would have missed meeting Sandy. She was the first to recommend "Anatomy of the Spirit." When I attended YLF a few weeks ago, I met my new bosom buddy Ilene. In our discussion she offered to loan me her Myss tapes and other spiritual tapes. And then, while watching daytime TV this week I saw Carolyn on the Oprah show. So you see, 3 messages were sent my way recently showing me I was meant to learn from her. She has a wonderful explanation of energy flow within our body and energy exchange with others and our universe. I have also discovered why I have struggled to be a better dancer. I can now see how I can apply what I am learning about the 7 Chakra's of the body to infuse my dance with a spiritual aspect that allows me to actually pray through body movement as the energy moves from one Chakrah to another. One of the things that attracted me to belly dance is its ritualistic form and its spiritual nature. Now I can actually pray with my body. Perhaps this is what was meant by the term "your body is your temple."

So, this has been one heck of a week for me. This "lull" of activity allowed me to spend more time "being" and learning and growing. I suggest to you that you make the time in your life to do the same. You don't know what you're missing. And to all of my friends who have strong spiritual lives, thank you for sharing them with me. Regardless of how we pray the fact that we do pray is the point. I now pray. [I can feel the breeze pick up now. No better time than now to ride the winds of change]

Spiritually yours,

cMc

p.s. You may go in peace to spread the words of the gospel. (can you tell I was raised Catholic?)

8/26/02—Cathy Update #14
(7 Weeks Post-Surgery, 18 Days After
1st AC Chemo Treatment)

Hair Today, Gone Tomorrow

I sit on the patio in Encinitas (not Encinada) with the ocean breeze blowing across my scalp. Talk about feeling free, although at night, I wear a cap 'cuz being bald gets cold. Yep. That inevitable moment has arrived.

I began the week by attending a "Look good, feel better" gathering at the Salon and Scalp Clinic I visited earlier. Mike offers his shop as host to other bosom buddies with the plan to help us learn how to fix ourselves up on the outside, which in turn may help us feel better on the inside. This program is a public service sponsored by the Cosmetic, Toilet and Fragrance Association Foundation, the American Cancer Society and the National Cosmetology Association. There we were, about a dozen bosom buddies, all sitting in a semi-circle chatting up a storm about who is getting what chemo treatments. How many days before your hair fell out? What lotion do you use for your dry skin? Where did you get your wig? Pass the cookies please. Oh my God, that's Katrina. I couldn't believe it. There she was, sitting across the room from me, wearing the same wig that I picked out for myself. We've known each other for almost 15 years, and I didn't know.

The strange thing about this breast cancer thing is that almost every single person I have told either has had it or knows someone who has had it. Cancer is so prevalent in our society today it is as if it's a part of life. And I mean LIFE, not death. So many survivors, so many stories that make my tumor seem like a pimple in comparison.

At the workshop we learned how to apply make up to cover the blotchy complexion that often comes with consuming chemo cocktails. Tips on how to draw in eyebrows and use eyeliner to replace the lashes that may fall out were high points for me. Some people lose their facial hair, some don't. Wigs and scarves may cover hair loss, but the facial hair is a tough one to hide. (If it goes, I just may go Joan Crawford with the eyebrows to see how many people cower in my presence. Perhaps it will help if I carry around a clothes hanger). We had such a strong bond at this gathering, almost like a support group, that there were times we drowned out the make up artist with our side conversations. We each received a box filled with free make up and skin care products from Estee Lauder, Avon, Lancome and other major brand cosmetics, all fit for our individual complexion color (light, med. dark and extra dark). Included is a booklet with tips for applying make up, skin care, scalp care and how to tie head scarves. Way cool! After two makeovers of volunteers from the audience, we learned hair tips from Mike. It is highly recommended that we shave our heads when the hair starts to fall out. Two reasons: 1. It's hard as hell to keep picking up all the stray hairs falling around the house, car, shower, where ever and 2. When we shave our head, we are the one in control, instead of waiting for it to fall out over time. (Being a control freak, I like the second reason best, but it was the hair falling out that prompted me to shave it since I am currently a guest in someone else's house. What a mess).

The day after the "Look good, feel better" workshop, my son Paul shaved his head. Scared the crap out of me when I saw him emerge from the bathroom. Then I realized, I just experienced the same shock that others may feel if they see me bald. Is this how it feels to be on the other side? It made me even more self-conscious about protecting others from seeing me bald. According to Mike, the average time for hair to grow back long enough and thick enough to give up the wig is about one year after it falls out. That's a long time to hide. *(When I returned home from my visit to Encinitas where I was writing this update, Paul had shaved his head knowing I was coming home bald. At our home, bald was the norm for quite some time)*

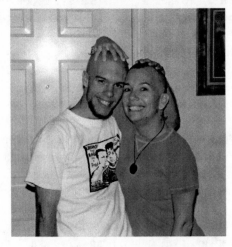

At home, bald was the norm!

I started feeling weak last week. Thought it strange, considering how good I felt right after my first chemo treatment. My blood results one week after chemo were actually better than they were before I began treatments. The normal range for blood tests are as follows:

white blood cell count (wbc) = 4k–10.8k cells per microliter
red blood cell count (rbc) = 4.2–5.4 million cells per microliter
hemoglobin (hgb) = 12–16 grams per dl
hematocrit (hema) = 37–47%
platelets = 133k–333k per microliter

One week after my first chemo treatment my counts were: wbc = 5.5; rbc = 4.25; hgb = 13.5; hema = 40.5; plate = 235; all within normal range. Two weeks after my first treatment, my wbc was way down to 2.0 and all others were down just a smidgen, but still normal. I also felt queasy enough to take two anti-nausea pills last week. My oncologist said it is normal that blood counts are lower two weeks after treatment but not one week after. Strange.

As you may have noticed by the first sentence of this e-mail, I am back in Encinitas (not Encinada). Charlie and I have returned to spend one last week near the ocean before summer ends. His friends, Henry, Joni and Hally from Illinois, have moved back to California and are now living in La Mesa. We visited their open house party on Saturday. There I met Helen, Joni's mom, a strong-willed, independent woman in her 60's, wearing her hair butch short and blond. She even complained it was too long (a whole inch) because she couldn't get in to see her hair stylist. I looked at her, knowing full well that I had only days left with my own hair, and admired her. She intentionally wears her hair extremely short. She couldn't give a damn what other people think about her. If only I could develop the same strong sense of self-esteem, perhaps I won't have to hide for a whole year. Meeting her made it easier for me to lose my hair.

The very next day I wrapped my hair in a scarf. It began to fall out slowly, as long as I didn't wash it. The follicles felt tingly, as if I had my hair up in a bun all day, then let it down to the point that my roots "ached." I knew it was time. On the drive back to Encinitas I was quite… contemplating… when will I shampoo my hair? Will it fall out in clumps? Should we shave it tonight or tomorrow? Thank heavens I was able to keep my hair until after the open house party. I'm gonna be bald tomorrow. Thank heavens I am surrounded by such wonderful friends, people who will understand that I am going to do this my way. This is going to be a celebration, 'cuz I'm not just going to shave my head, I'm gonna go PUNK first!

As my hair fell out by the handful when I showered, I cried. I allowed myself to grieve, for the next step is acceptance and the ritual of shaving my head, my way! I have been prepared for this moment for weeks, gathering punk apparel from my son's friends and keeping it with me at all times. I announced to Charlie, Dennis and Katie that tonight's the night. We'll shave my head while watching "Six Feet Under" (one of my favorite HBO programs, not that I plan to be there any time soon). But first I had to get ready…on with the black shirt with zippers and silver studs, spiked bracelet and a leather necklace with spikes and miniature handcuffs…then, thick black eye liner, dark red eye shadow, and black lipstick. A bat earring on one side and a safety pin on the other. I had to look the part if I'm gonna have a Mohawk before I go bald. What better time than now, what better excuse than this. Charlie snapped away with his camera as Katie did the deed with the clippers. I must admit, punk does not look good at the age of 41. The wrinkles are totally out of place, but it did make the ritual fun. I sported my Mohawk for about 30 minutes. When the Mohawk was gone, and nothing but nubs were left on my head, I felt good. I felt cleansed.

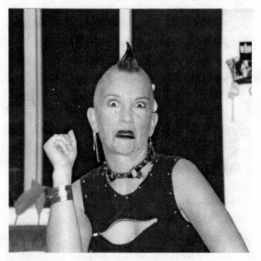

When I sent this picture out with my e-mail update for that week,
people really got scared.

There is a part of me that is glad the hair is gone. I had 15 years of history hanging from my head when I was first diagnosed. That's a lot of baggage. Now, many cells in and on my body are relatively new. I have dumped my past so it should be easier for me to live in the present. Interesting concept.

I love the hat I wear around the house. It's so comfortable. I wore my wig into town today. Itchy, but stylish. I have several scarves to tie into turbans so I have lots of different "looks" I can try. The big change will be returning to work, looking so different than before. Helen, give me strength. The disability insurance company is pushing. They want me back to work as soon as possible. I had to call them to push it back one week as they wanted me back to work the Monday after my next treatment. Physically I think I can handle it, if I return part time. Mentally, I'm gonna have to see just how long I can handle wearing the wig before I rip it off my head and throw it at someone in a meeting. (Gee, that isn't very optimistic thinking is it). I don't know if I have enough Irish blood in me to go Sinead O'Conner at work. I should feel "in style" with the popularity of Dr. Evil and Mini-Me, they even have a new Rap video. There is even a car commercial on TV where a girl wears different wigs with each functional change of the car, then pops back into view… bald, saying "change is a good thing." Besides, the first card in my totem is the eagle, a sign of leadership. Let's make that a bald eagle. Maybe I could sell carnations at the airport. Now I'm ranting.

This is gonna take some time getting used to. Otherwise, I count my blessings I feel so good.

Until next time,

cMc

p.s. It's fine with me if you sh-hair this with others.

77

9/2/02—Cathy Update #15
(8 Weeks Post-Surgery, 4 Days After
2nd AC Chemo Rreatment)

Cathy's Glamour Tips

I tried wearing the wig several times this past week. Until it gets "worn in" I think it will feel itchy, and if I don't wear it because it feels itchy, it will never get "worn in." Life likes to throw us a Catch 22 now and then. *(Eventually I discovered a gel filled wig liner that made wig wearing comfortable. I also learned many scarf and hat tricks to reduce the time I wore wigs)*

When I purchased my wig I also bought a light blue cotton cap (adorable), a mauve silk scarf and a sleep cap to keep my head warm. Must have options for all occasions. While we were driving home from Encinitas (not Encinada) we stopped at our favorite pit stop the Willow Ranch Bar BQ in Buttonwillow. Great food. Now, I was overly concerned about my looks because this was the first time I was "out in public" without my wig. I chose to wear my light blue cotton cap since it was casual enough to wear with my blue jeans. It was at least 100 degrees outside and as I walked through the front door of the restaurant my eyes focused on the reflection of the two ladies who had just passed me as they left the building. I watched the reflection of their eyes to see if they were looking back at me and wondering why I would be wearing a hat on such a hot day. My focus on them was so intent I never saw my own reflection. Whew, they didn't even glance at me. As with most motorists, I sped past the waitress at the cash register and made a B-line for the restroom. I walked into the stall and locked the door. I was safe. No one else was in the restroom. When I was done, I walked out of the stall and rounded the corner and came face to face with the mirror. There it was…to my horror… right in the middle of my forehead… the produce sticker I had peeled off the apple and stuck to my forehead while we were in the car. I completely forgot about it. I DIED LAUGHING. Here I am trying to be inconspicuous so that no one notices I have no hair and guess what, no one notices. What they may notice is a silly woman walking around with a produce sticker on her forehead. Lesson in maturity. (Cathy glamour tip #1.)

I had an incredible outpour of support from all of you last week. I guess my last update sounded a bit sad, but that was not my intent. As you can see, all things work out for the best (or in my life, the funniest) over time. I have been showered with jewels lately. They include a hand made glass bead bracelet with a breast cancer ribbon designed right into the bead and hand made jewelry from our dear friends who have a Venetian glass bead company. I make noise with all the bangles I wear, which is a treat for a sign language interpreter 'cuz we can't usually wear large and noisy jewelry. I received 4 post cards from a bosom buddy visiting Scotland. Someone even left me a voice mail message at work, not knowing I was out on disability, and offered to "kiss it and make it feel better." He obviously didn't know the location of my surgery. Your words of support this past week have helped a lot. Thank you so very much.

While in Encinitas (not Encinada), Charlie and I visited the Self-Realization Fellowship, founded by Paramahansa Yogananda. (Most of the time I can't remember his name, so I call him Parmesana YogiBera) Founded in 1920, this organization strives to spread his teachings of prayer through yoga and metaphysical meditations. The grounds at the fellowship are gorgeous with gardens reaching to the edge of cliffs overlooking the ocean. It is a beautifully serene place to sit in solitude and pray. It was especially comforting to me the day after my Mohawk incident. I fit right in here, as some of the disciples there don't have any hair either (envision a Buddhist monk). This is another visit on my continued spiritual journey to involve more prayer in my life.

Thursday was my second chemo treatment and we had a full house. Ses was busy as ever tending to 6 patients. I didn't put a henna tattoo around Cathy-ter this week because of the Mohawk incident, so I did the next best thing. A bindi is a decoration placed in the middle of women's foreheads in East Indian cultures, much like the produce sticker which is used in the US. I placed a circle of gold and black bindis in a design around Cathy-ter. It shimmered in the sunlight and was quite beautiful. (Cathy glamour tip #2) Ses had me model for all the other patients at the chemo lounge and called the doctor in to see. He is East Indian and the first thing he said was, "I have to show my wife." Another day of chemo, without a hitch, just the way I like it.

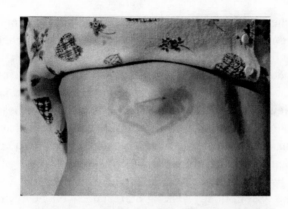

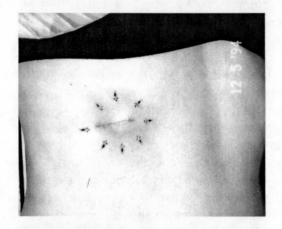

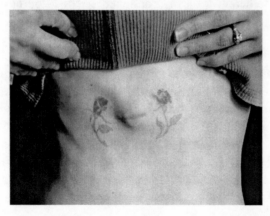

A few of my Cathy-ter decorations: henna, bindis and rub on tattoos.

Next new public viewing challenge…the Scottish Games. I was worried that I wouldn't feel up to attending the games this year, being only 3 days after my chemo treatment. I was determined not to allow these treatments to prevent me from participating in my regular annual life events. We have a long standing family tradition of attending the games every year and if I could come up with a way to attend and still be comfortable, it would be done. For those of you who don't know, McClain is a Scottish name. Every year thousands of Scots gather at the Pleasanton fairgrounds on the hottest weekend of the year to throw cabers (phone poles), eat haggis (don't ask), dance and play bag pipes. Of course, many other things happen, too many to list here. My good buddy Bob, Charlie, Paul and I start out early with a swig (or 2 or 3) of single malt scotch, then head to the gathering and games for a day of heritage. (Thanks to the chemo drugs I was able to take a few nips of 16 yr. old scotch) I knew it would be hot and I would get tired, so I borrowed a wheelchair so I wouldn't have to walk great distances. Hello!! If you haven't thought of this one, do it. I don't care what ails you, use a wheelchair and you will be able to enjoy many events. I wore my mauve silk scarf under a straw hat with my floral dress that matched our family tartan sash. (Cathy glamour tip #3) The silk scarf was light and airy and the straw hat was a good sun block. The wheelchair is also a great way to carry all the tokens I collected throughout the day, including the new head scarf I purchased. I noticed throughout the day that people didn't really even look at me. I thought being in a wheelchair would draw more attention than it did. I guess we have the Americans with Disabilities Act to thank for inviting people with disabilities to be a part of our landscape so we don't even notice them as outsiders. (Besides, hanging out with Bob, I'm certain that all attention goes to him and his boisterous antics. This year he sang the Sponge Bob Square Pants song out loud while waiting in line for bangers and mash. And people sang along.)

One of the most phenomenal events at these Scottish Games is the massed bands. I know it's hard to handle bag pipes if it isn't in your blood, but if it is…you'll never be the same after hearing over 600 bagpipes playing "Amazing Grace" in unison. I usually cry a bit when I hear it, but this year, the tears streamed down my face. "I once was lost, but now I'm found. Was blind but now I see." I was surrounded by my family, aunts, uncles, parents, brothers, nieces, my good buddy Bob, Charlie and Paul. It was quite emotional. And damn, I looked good.

As we were leaving in the afternoon, rolling out into the parking lot, I felt a sense of accomplishment. I didn't feel as self-conscious any more. People didn't stare at me all day, they didn't even notice me. I am not the center of other people's universe, so get over it. All this preoccupation with what other's think about how I look, it's so shallow. As we got in the car, I noticed Paul had put a baseball cap on top of my straw hat. We wheeled out of the stadium, across the parking lot, all that distance, and I was wearing two hats. (Cathy glamour tip #4) So you see, no matter how hard I may try to be glamorous, it's not always my call.

cMc

9/8/02—Cathy Update #16
(2 Months Post-Surgery, 10 Days After
2nd AC Chemo Treatment)

Working the Arm

I'm sitting in the Garden of Eden again, contemplating the week in review. This is such an incredible space, our own little Self-Realization garden, right here in Paradise. We did outdoor projects this weekend to take advantage of my current strength. It seems that 6-12 days after my chemo treatments are my best days, so I try to make my plans accordingly. I am returning to work part time tomorrow (25%-avg. 10 hrs/week). We have many important events coming up and my heart pulls me back to the office. I love my job and my loyalty to my clients (I prefer the word constituency, but they didn't vote) is one of my weaknesses. Don't worry, as many of my bosom buddies have warned, I plan to take it easy and will not attempt anything beyond my healing needs.

I began physical therapy last Wednesday. In doing my arm stretching exercises (climbing the walls, literally) I noticed extremely tight strands under my left arm pit. I wanted to borrow a guitar pick from Paul to see if I can play out a tune, the strands were so tight. I thought it was tendons and for a while, they hurt when I stretched, all the way past my elbow. *(To be honest, I was not vigilant with my arm exercises, and I paid the price. Do not follow my example. Faithfully do your exercises every day, or you will regret it. Fortunately, I improved my exercise regime and I am better today, but my arm still tightens up every now and then)* According to Carla, my physical therapist (another great personality to brighten my path), these are the remnants of my lymphatic system in my arm. One of my bosom buddies experienced the same thing. She said, "one day, I reached out, and "snap," the strings broke, and the tightness was gone *(hasn't happened to me yet)*. Someone explained the lymphatic system to me this way. It's like a string of old Christmas tree lights, when one light bulb is burned out, the rest of them go out too. Since I had 2 nodes removed from one zone, and 3 from another, it is likely that 2 of my lymphatic cluster systems are now dead. This will effect the drainage of my arm all the way down pass my elbow. I hope there are enough other lymph systems in my arm to effectively avoid developing lymphedema (every interpreter's nightmare).

Carla has shown me some new exercises, less aggressive yet more effective. She is also massaging my scar tissue (mmmmm, with cocoa butter) to break it down and help alleviate tightness caused by excessive tissue buildup. I was doing tissue massage myself, but my technique was all wrong. I highly recommend to fellow bosom buddies to learn how to do your exercises and tissue massage right from the start. Consult with a physical therapist BEFORE surgery so you won't do any damage using the wrong technique. It's not enough to try learning from drawings and text on paper, demonstration is much more effective.

Needless to say (never worked on me, I always say it anyway), I will have extremely light interpreting duty when I return to work. Fortunately, there is always enough disability services work to keep me busy a mere 25% time. My interpreting is limited to administrative (non-technical) topics, no more than 30 minutes consecutive, and no group discussions (group dialogue goes too fast). I have been fortunate, and many tell me similar experiences, that my doctor lets me decide my limitations. No one other than another sign language interpreter could possibly know more than I would about the physical and mental stresses of interpreting to be able to determine my work restrictions. I discussed these limitations with my co-worker and team interpreter, Sheila. She agreed that they seemed reasonable.

Sign language interpreting is often misunderstood. Many believe that signing and interpreting are the same. They think if you know sign language, you can also interpret. Well, it's true you must know sign language FLUENTLY in order to be able to interpret, but the process of interpreting is an additional skill and physically and mentally more demanding. I sometimes explain it the following way, although there is no scientific basis in my perspective. When interpreting, the mind is processing information in such a way that the muscles (neck, shoulders, arms, wrists) are "bathed" in stress. I could sign all day, and never feel fatigue, but I can only interpret for one hour straight (depending on conditions) before actual pain can begin. I'm from the old school. There were no safety standards when I began interpreting at the ripe old age of 17. I would interpret for hours without a break, and thus, have developed a mild case of carpel tunnel syndrome and tendonitis. Today, preventing a flare up is essential, and this is why we have such a rigid structure to our interpreting safety standards.

Any assignment longer than one hour is often teamed by two interpreters. I work in a scientific research laboratory and at my work place some meetings are so difficult and fast we team even one-hour assignments. There are no signs for much of our technical vocabulary, so finger spelling or inventing signs are necessary. In the past 22 years, my Deaf colleagues and I have invented over 400 signs that are used at at our site only. Speed is a constant problem in this scientific environment. I truly believe that as our media experiences bombard us with information at such high rates of speed, it is affecting the speed in which people actually talk. I observe that the younger scientists and engineers speak more rapidly than the older ones. I have invented the label of "speed-talking-mumbler" to describe to other interpreters some working conditions related to certain clients's co-workers. Add to that, the intensity of a group discussion, with people interrupting each other (double time for interpreters), and the complexity of transcribing in your mind "ok…what is the sign language equivalent for that English word?…oh…there is none…how do I spell that?" This mental process must happen in a micro-second (and chemo-brain slows me down). I would estimate some of our technical group meetings average over 300 words per minute. We have some of the most difficult interpreting conditions that exist, and we have some of the best sign language interpreters in the state of California working for us. For this reason, I must refrain from strenuous interpreting until I am fully able to do so and trust our other interpreters to handle the load (I don't want to be responsible by making mistakes that lead to someone failing in their job).

One lesson I learned in my cancer experience is that my work place did not shut down when I left. In the past 22 years, I have missed probably no more than 10 interpreting assignments. An interpreter simply cannot cancel last minute without extreme guilt pangs. You can't just ring up another interpreter with 3 hours notice for a replacement. This resource is just too scarce. Handing over my interpreting responsibilities (especially classified assignments, of which only 2 other interpreters can do) was the toughest part of being gone. But everyone survived. (Everyone, not everything. My budget suffered having to pay outside interpreters to replace me. Maybe now they will see just how valuable I am and pay me more. Oh, that's right, I forgot. Money doesn't mean that much to me any more (shhh, don't tell the boss). It is a relief to be able to let go of my old sense of having it all on my shoulders. Why do we do such cruel things to ourselves? So go ahead, take vacation, the world won't stop revolving just because you need a break!

In preparation for returning to work, I am trying to re-establish a routine. I haven't worn a watch in 2 months. *(I still don't wear one to this day)* How wonderful is that!? In addition to getting up earlier, trying to exercise (if I'm up to it) and putting on make up in the mornings, I have set aside 9-10:00 PM as my "spiritual hour," reserved (uninterrupted) for reading about spirituality and attempting to learn how to meditate. I may extend that period of time as time goes on, as I don't want to stop the attention I have given to this part of my life. I also have a collection of hats and scarves so I should have plenty of fashion options. (Because our hands flail in the air, interpreters are always the center of attention. It's hard to get this perception out of my mind that everyone is looking at me). I found a wonderful accessory to help make wearing my wig more comfortable. It is a gel-filled strap called the "Comfy Grip" that I bought from Marzel's in Pleasanton. Now I can wear my wig for hours without itching.

Speaking of fashion, I had another fashion revelation this week. As the weather begins to cool down, one morning at 2:00 AM I woke up with a cold head (Not a head cold. A cold head. Hair is a wonderful insulator). I bought a sleep cap but wasn't prepared to use it, so I searched, half asleep, trying to find it. I finally gave up, putting a pair of underwear on my head, and going back to sleep (You may laugh, but it worked!). Now, this is not a bikini, and I don't own any thong underwear, we are talking Granny underwear plenty large enough to cover my entire head. Charlie laughed out loud when I told him, saying he could see me walking out of the house in the morning to get the newspaper with underwear on my head. So perhaps I should begin a new line of cancer fashions, including underwear hats, produce sticker bindis and henna tattoos. Heaven knows what else may come to mind during my experience. I still have 6 more months to go until my treatments (chemo and radiation) are done. Plenty of time for my sick and twisted mind to invent more fashion trends.

My mom and I went to the lunch and the movies this week to see "My Big Fat Greek Wedding." You gotta see it! This is the first time in 10 years my mom has gone to the movie theatre. The last time she went was to take my son Paul to see "Robin Hood, Men in Tights." She doesn't watch much TV, and when she does, it is usually PBS, so she had quite a media culture-shock sitting through the previews. I just love the fact that I am spending so much more time with her these days. (When was the last time you called your mom to say "I love you?") Just before we left the house, I discovered another friend who has cancer. Paul was out front, and I could hear a stranger's voice saying "tell your mom that Cupcake is here." My most, bestest, favorite guard from the Lab is Michael, nicknamed Cupcake. He is short, with dark hair and cute as a bug, with one of the most pleasant personalities I have ever had the pleasure to know. Mike walked up to me, with some kind of a device hanging from his shoulder, gave me a big hug and said, "as soon as I found out about your cancer, I had to come see you." He was so concerned about me. How do I feel? How am I handling this? Never once did he mention what he was going through, not until I noticed how much weight he lost and asked why. He has colon cancer, and it spread to his stomach. He is currently receiving chemotherapy 24/7 (5-Fu) through that device he wears like a purse hanging on his shoulder. He is undergoing daily radiation treatments as well, to shrink the tumor before surgery next month. He will follow with further chemotherapy and radiation post-surgery. It is hoped that the stomach tumors go away with treatments, as at this time, surgery is not expected to help. He will undergo a complete colonostomy and will need to wear a colonostomy bag the rest of his life. In his own words, "I don't care, as long as I get to be with my children as long as I can, that's what's important." He has such an incredible attitude and spirit. He was more interested in making sure I was alright than in talking about his experience. Seeing him that day renewed my appreciation for how good I have it. Compared to him, I had cancer-lite. Looking at the photos and reading through a book gifted to me from my friend David, "ART.RAGE.US. a collection of art and writings from breast cancer survivors," I am once again face to face with just how lucky I am to be experiencing so little problems.

I want to thank all of you too, for I truly believe that the prayers you send on a regular basis fuel the healing energy that lines my path with gold bricks. (can you tell we worked on repairing the brick patio yesterday?)

Gotta stop! I can't believe how long winded (long fingered?) I am with these updates.

Love,

cMc

p.s. go ahead and tell on me, I dare you.

9/15/02—Cathy Update #17
(10 Weeks Post-Surgery, 3 Days Before
3rd AC Chemo Treatment)

I'm Fine!

Love,

cMc

p.s. We deserve a break today, you from reading and me from writing. Stay tuned next week for more relentless ramblings.... same Cat time, same Cat channel.

9/22/02—Cathy Update #18
(11 Weeks Post-Surgery, 4 Days After
3rd AC Chemo Treatment)

The Benefits of Benefits: Ode to an Employer

(This update may upset some readers. Not everyone is blessed to have great medical benefits, let alone good benefits or any at all. If you are one such individual, please skip this update. I don't want to rub in how lucky I am to have something you don't have. I do, however, want to remind others who are as fortunate as I that they have a good thing and should appreciate it while they have it).

Never before have I come to appreciate so much in my life. This week my employer, celebrates its 50th anniversary. No better time than now to express my appreciation for how my healing has been supplemented by the nurturing of a community of coworkers and an institution that give its employees so much more than many realize. I truly believe my speedy recovery is aided by my lack of worries about finances due to the incredible benefits provided to me here.

I returned to work part time on September 9 in hopes of contributing to my position as I felt only I could. I am one of the fortunate few who not only have a job, but a vocation, a calling, something so much more than just a pay check. I just finished my third chemotherapy treatment last Thursday, 3 down and 5 to go. I guess working part time took more of a toll than I thought, as I spent 3 days straight in bed after my treatment, sleeping off the past two weeks of extra effort. This is not a complaint, it does feel good to get back involved at work. Our "Family Days" plans and the 50th anniversary celebration needed some of my attention. I returned just in time to interpret for former Senator and astronaut John Glenn last Wednesday. (A local columnist even wrote a story about his visit to the presentation and he mentioned me by name in the article regarding my interpreting, what a hoot!) There is no hiding I am back to work. A few other timely projects need to get underway and with Disabilities Awareness Week coming up in October, I need to know we are well prepared. Don't forget the Special Olympics Walk for the Gold on October 5!

I returned to work well prepared. Thanks to dear Donna (remember that 'community' I told you about). I found a platter full of fresh fruit, cheese, bread and juice waiting for me in my office when I arrived. I brought in a foam cushion for sleeping so I can take a nap in the middle of the day. I learned, however, that in order to be a hard core napper, I needed more amenities. So I now have a sheet, blanket, ear plugs, eye covers, a sleep cap and socks. It'll take an earthquake to wake me from my nap now. I have such a wimpy work schedule, a full 8 hours one week followed by 12 hours the next. My work-day consists of 2 hours of work, followed by 2 hours for lunch and a nap, followed by 2 more hours of work. Wow, I don't now how I make it through the day. Once you fill in the phone calls and e-mails while I am at home, it does add up to more than a 25% work schedule, but whose counting? I guess the disability insurance company could be, perhaps.

I am able to return to work thanks to a program called Stay at Work/Return to Work, offered by University of California and Liberty Mutual disability insurance. This offers me a chance to work enough to contribute, but not work so much as to have any negative impact on my health. If I were to remain on disability full time, I could only earn 70% of my usual paycheck, but with this program, I can return to work part time and earn up to 100% of my usual paycheck. I can also retain all my other benefits as long as my work hours average 50% over the course of the past 12 months. Way cool! I consider this a great balance on my road to recovery. *(I never did see 100% of my paycheck, but I firmly believe returning to work part time at a job I love helped me heal faster)*

Oh, did I ask you yet? Do you have supplemental disability insurance? Yes? Good! No? Wassa matta wit you? I don't care what your excuse is, get some kind of disability insurance. Don't think of it as, "how much will this cost me each month?" think of it as, "how much peace of mind is this going to give me if or when I get seriously ill?" You can't put a price on peace of mind. Even if you have to pick 30 day or 180 day waiting periods for your insurance, do it! I have seen my employer's Catastrophic Leave Program supply employees with enough leave donations to make up the difference during their waiting periods. This is an incredible benefit you can't afford to overlook. Remember, people with disabilities refer to everyone else as T.A.B... Temporarily Able Bodied. In our lifetime, 90% of us will acquire a permanent or temporary disability. Believe me, I'm in the business, I know what I'm talking about. Thanks to the benefits this single mom has chosen, my son will be able to enjoy his senior year in high school because my lifestyle hasn't changed due to my temporary disability. Senior pictures, cap and gown, Disneyland trip, just to name a few, no problem!

That is just the tip of the iceberg. My hospital bill for two surgeries = $34,177.78; surgeon for two surgeries = $3611; $1540 x 8 for chemotherapy treatments; $120 x 15 for check ups and blood work; 30 radiation treatments to go and I have no idea how much each of the pre-tests I already had were. I won't be surprised of we end up near $100,000 by the time the calculator battery dies. And how much do I pay for my medical benefits each month out of my paycheck? $000.00 (I don't claim this is all perfect, as I did spend time this past week following up on mis-billed invoices. It is important to double check and be very friendly with your benefits coordinator, she can make your life easier or cause you severe heartburn. Remember…a spoon full of sugar. But believe me, the price is right and the effort is worth it to make sure your credit report stays clean.)

Moral to the story? I must admit, I too have fallen into the trap of complaining about wages, especially at this time of year when everyone is moaning about performance appraisals. (For those of you who are not my coworkers, simply apply this lecture to your own place of work, or, if you are self employed, just smile) One of the benefits of working here is longevity. Those of us here long enough to be stuck in the old salary structure are also lucky enough to still be here, but unlucky enough to be stuck in the old salary structure (feel a loop?). While many fled for dot com heaven, they came crawling back years later. Some of us stuck it out and took advantage of other benefits, such as tuition reimbursement. Did I tell you? While I got 6 hours off per week paid leave to attend classes at one of the most expensive universities in California, my employer paid my tuition. Thank you very much to a total of $38,000 and a BA in Communication from University of the Pacific. In 1998 and again in 2001 I participated in Survey Action Teams that evaluated employee's comments from two surveys we conducted here. While many employees complained about salaries, only a few recognized how fortunate we are to work for an employer who offers such incredible benefits. You may choose not to take advantage of the benefits offered to you, but that does not erase the fact that they are there for the taking. Look deeper!

I find myself in a situation now where I look deeper than the paycheck. I don't look this gift horse in the mouth. I look it in the eye with pride. I look at what I do and I enjoy it. I look around the office and I like the people I work with. They feel like family, heck, I like some of them better than some of my family (not you mom!). I appreciate the benefits. Geez Louise, I just bought a new cellular phone and changed my phone plan. When I mentioned where I work, they gave me 15% off all accessories and 5% off my monthly phone bill. I didn't even ask for it, it just happened.

For today, realize there are a lot of benefits to your job, to your life, to your planet…if you take the time to look…deeper.

9/30/02—Cathy Update #19
(12 Weeks Post-Surgery, 12 Days After 3rd AC Chemo Treatment)

Fried Eggs and Toast

I have been experiencing some side effects from chemotherapy that I read about during my research on this matter. I wondered if I would experience them, as some people do and some don't. I have been fortunate to experience them mildly so I haven't even mentioned them so far.

For the past several weeks I have had a dull ache in my lower back. Ovary-ache is my suspicion as many pre-menopausal chemo patients go through what they call "oblation" of the ovaries. Sounds like an omelet, and it basically is. The ovaries get "scrambled" as the chemo does its damage. I much prefer to think that my eggs are actually being "fried" and when someone asks me, "How are you doing?" I like to respond, "fried eggs, thank you." If I am having a particularly weary day, I respond, "fried eggs and toast." This oblation process can lead to menopause, which I anticipate with much joy. If I have to go through menopause eventually, I much prefer to go through it now when I am working part-time. I doubt I will be able to use menopause as an excuse in the future to take disability time off, and that is a shame, as some women really suffer through it. The irony of all this is I just can't seem to do enough to prevent getting pregnant. I had a tubal ligation 6 years ago, then after suffering miserable periods years later, I went back on birth control pills. Those are the very pills that I suspect expedited the growth of my breast tumor and brought to light its presence. So after having both a tubal and taken birth control pills, I am now frying my ovaries, just to make darn sure I ain't having any more kids. I am lucky as I don't want any more children. Some young breast cancer patients aren't so lucky. I read an article in Rosie magazine this week about a woman who had surgery and some chemo "during" her pregnancy. There are several great articles about breast cancer in that October 2002 issue and it is worth reading.

Another side effect I have been experiencing is dehydration and the loss of mucus production. Chemotherapy effects fast growing cells in the body and mucus is one of them. In addition to drinking (attempting to remember to) a gallon of water each day, I discovered some over the counter products that help. Biotene gum helps to activate saliva glands to whet my whistle and Stoppers 4 dry mouth spray is just one of the products on the market with enzymes to re-hydrate the mucus linings of the mouth. I keep a bottle next to my bed as I tend to sleep with my mouth open and night time is when I dry out the worst. I also use a humidifier to keep the air in my bedroom more moist. I also notice that doing deep breathing exercises (mostly as a novice meditator) is difficult as my lungs are not as comfortable expanding so much with a dryer lining. The most important issue for me to watch for is thrush (a white fungal growth on the tongue). It is common for chemo patients to develop thrush in their mouth due to reduced mucus and inability to fight off infection. I need to keep excellent oral hygiene, and try as I might, I can't seem to brush my teeth after every meal. I do brush, floss, use a water pik and mouthwash (without alcohol) every night. So far so good.

Enough about being a patient. I prefer to write about the 30th annual San Francisco Blues Festival where Charlie and I spent this past weekend. This event marks an important change in my life that has all come about thanks to this cancer gig. I didn't go because I have the Blues, I went because, as Steve Miller so adequately put it in his opening song, "I've got to let the good times roll." Although I must admit some of the songs did fit my mood, particularly when Elvin Bishop and the boys sang, "I'll be glad when I've got my groove back again." I used to hate going to these things, but now I see and appreciate the annual event as a ritual of celebration. I used to be such an impatient person that I thought sitting around all weekend listening to music was an incredible waste of time. Must be "doing"…didn't know how to "be" still long enough to soak it in. I used to go to this event because Charlie is a huge Blues fan. It felt like an obligation to me and I whined about the cold (or the heat) or whatever I could find to complain about while I was there. This year I saw it through a different pair of eyes, and oh what a beautiful weekend it was.

Festival culture is an anthropological gold mine. People arrive early in line to socialize and attempt to be the first "blanket runner" to claim their turf of the unclaimed territory in front of the stage. There are unspoken rules of order regarding blanket real estate loans (putting your blanket down on the grass to claim your turf) and rights to air space from eye-view to mid-stage.

No one dare move your blanket once it is placed, even if you leave it there for hours, empty of chairs and bodies, it still cannot be moved. These neighborhoods of blanket dwellers have pathways designed by civil engineers who have been drinking beer since getting in line at 8:00 in the morning (some earlier, some stronger than beer). Walking through these neighborhoods requires patience and the ability to step over obstacles, as maps will do you no good in the ever-changing pathways to the porta-potties.

The consistent cast of characters we see once each year is as colorful as the hats and attire you would expect, especially at a San Francisco outdoor event. Michael and Jess, our dear friends who attend various Blues festivals with us, meet us in line early in the morning for socializing, breakfast and mimosas (latte for me). This year, as in the past, Jess presents me with some beautiful creation of jewelry, a pearl bracelet she made. Thanks Jess! Michael brings his red wagon with 4WD wheels so we don't have to carry all our junk in and can have enough gear to satisfy any need during the day. We bump into Ozel and her mother Floe while in line, by far the most fashionable festival gear in town (hand woven picnic basket and beautiful bags). They have been attending this festival every year since its inception 30 years ago. Seeing them makes this feel like we are at a reunion and I look forward to future festivals when I can say, "I made it to another one, with my health and happiness intact." Many faces are familiar and others are known for their unique presence, like the couple who bring a 5' x 5' dance floor and jitter bug through the day. And don't forget the man I call "Free Willy" (name changed to protect privacy) who wears a colorful cotton poncho and we are all sure has absolutely nothing underneath, except his free Willy.

The food is as diverse as the neighborhoods of blanket dwellers. In addition to what you expect (fried whatever, beer and wine) there is a delicious menu including jambalaya from the Gingerbread House, chicken and 3 flavors of cornbread stuffing from Stuffedbird, peach cobbler, Indian cuisine, Gyros sandwiches, BBQ oysters, Bavarian roasted nuts, Ben and Jerry's ice cream, Tri-tip and a full service bar, to name a few. Vendors selling clothing, hats, sunglasses, jewelry, and wares complete the scene all with a backdrop of the Palace of Fine Arts, San Francisco bay and the Golden Gate Bridge with sailboats floating underneath. How could I have been so ungrateful in the past, not appreciating this view of humanity, dancing to the music, enjoying the sunshine, and celebrating life?

For me the festival was a great opportunity to display hat and scarf fashion. Believe me, living in Tracy it is difficult to dress up my head fancy without stares. Tracy (my town) isn't known for high fashion and hat wear consists mostly of cowboy hats. I have always been fashion-impaired as I never took time in the past to worry much about how I looked. The "fashion accessory" gene passed down to me from my ancestors (who believed looking good meant more than paying the bills), has long been dormant. But this weekend I was on my great-aunt Clara's turf, San Francisco, where she was famous in the 40's and 50's for wearing beautiful hats, gloves and fashion (although my memories of her include her slip always showing, even when she wore a sari). I guess you could say she had great "hatitude." Aunt Clara was my guardian angel this weekend and, if I do say so myself, I looked "mawvelous dawling." I chose not to wear my wig for several reasons. It's uncomfortable to wear a wig with a hat, I don't get enough chances to wear the scarves, and to be quite honest, I just don't like the feel of the wig. Artificial hair and elastic feels unnatural against my skin and I can only stand it for about 4 hours. Besides, a festival is a place where people want to let their hair down. I chose to take my hair off! Wearing a scarf under my hat became quite a blessing as I was able to block the scorching sun from my face with a quick flip and tuck of the scarf under my hat. As the temperatures cooled down, the scarf kept my neck warm and it was a great way to cover the ear plugs in my ears (We interpreters need to protect our hearing). Future festivals will not be complete without a scarf under my hat!

I completed the weekend with a new addition to my charm bracelet, a small guitar to represent this year's SF Blues Festival (I started a charm bracelet with the cross blessed by the Pope and have added to it through each significant event of my cancer journey). A symbol of my new found ability to sit still long enough to take in all the wonders of blues festival culture and to participate with my fellow blanket dwellers in this annual ritual of celebration. Life is good!

Love,

cMc

p.s. share the gift of gab with my blessings.

10/7/02—Cathy Update #20
(3 Months Post-Surgery, 2 Days Before
4th AC Chemo Treatment)

Dare to Dream

After my last treatment I slept constantly for 3 days straight. No matter how good it may feel at the time, don't do that. I paid the price by not being able to sleep at night for almost a week afterward. I tried all my tried and true remedies, such as chamomile tea and a hot bath before bedtime. Listening to meditation tapes while lying in bed didn't help either as my mind kept wondering off. During this phase in my life where I don't expend much physical energy, my mind tends to keep going at it's normal fast pace and in order to knock it out at night, my body needs to be tired enough to counter act the brain race. I am now focusing on following a more routine schedule, getting up early every day, doing my arm and leg exercises, doing more chores (going to work helps) and taking only a brief nap during the day. Keeping busy is helping to make me tired enough to fall asleep at night. Believe me, this staying home thing can sure get you out of whack on following a routine. Sleeping for 10 hours every night is sure easy to do, but not really necessary for me at this stage.

One of the problems with sleeping was my constant day dreaming (I would call it night dreaming but that would imply I was asleep) about our Paradise home after the remodel. Before all this cancer stuff came about, Charlie and I were deep into planning a huge remodel project. Everything was put on hold and I haven't thought about it at all until recently when I began talking again with our architect, my friend Dennis. I get so darn excited about this that I can't stop thinking about it when I lay my head on the pillow at night. We have been planning this remodel for 5 years and we are counting down the months now before the project begins *(ha! I should have said years, not months)*. I truly believe having this dream to look forward to has also helped my healing process. I have a lot to live for and I'm going to see this remodel through if it kills me. So, what can an anal-retentive, obsessive compulsive girl do at night to keep her mind busy when she can't sleep? Build a model of the finished house project! No cardboard box is sacred. Where's the masking tape? Gotta buy some rubber cement and new razor blades for the box cutter. Watch out, hell hath no fury like Cathy when she's hunkered down on a project.

While in the craft store shopping for razor blades I ran into my next door neighbor Mary and her son Brian. They were shopping for materials to build a model of a California mission, a typical 4th grade project in our town. I realized, there I was, 41 years old, acting like a 4th grader, building my little model of our dream house, and loving every minute of it. It's a good thing I inherited my Dad's genes for meticulously building models. I remember him working for hours in the garage building his remote control airplanes out of balsa wood and fine plastic sheets. Later he earned his pilot's license and had his own plane (he called it Tweedy Bird). He saw his dream come true. Later I plan to live in our dream house represented by this model, and I can't die for at least 20 years because that is how long it's going to take to finish all the work that needs to be done. This is my carrot dangling in front of me. Motivation to keep healthy.

Some people have asked me if I have thought about death since my diagnosis, and to be perfectly honest, that has never crossed my mind. (My outlook of survival is the reason I don't talk much about death in my updates). I was more hung up on losing my hair and feeling sick from the chemo. It is not my destiny to die from this cancer, we caught it early enough and are treating it thoroughly. My mother is doing wonderfully 16 years post diagnosis, so no, I never even considered that death was an option here. I'll probably die from the bleeding ulcer that may develop when I plan to move into the Paradise house and we still have no roof from the construction project. Nah! The true test of my new stress reduced life style will be this remodel project. I have become so much more patient and accepting of mishaps and errors since this cancer thing, I hope I can bring that with me into this remodel project. I'm sure the contractor would also appreciate the new attitude.

Meanwhile, I have returned to sleeping at night, and never slept more soundly than Saturday after our 3 mile 'Walk for the Gold' for the Special Olympics. Thank you to all of the people who donated time and money. Our team of 10 walkers raised over $1300 and enjoyed a pleasant stroll through Pleasanton. We were prepared for anything. Our motley crew included Chemo Cathy, my saintly mother and her bad back, one walker who has two titanium hips and another who injured her foot the day before. I brought my trusty wheelchair in case I grew tired or my mother's back started causing problems, but we had many walkers who could benefit from the care-chair (I highly recommend to my bosom buddies on chemo or radiation, don't avoid participating in events you enjoy! If you feel tired, rent a wheelchair for a mere $10 a day and enjoy your life. You'll be surprised to learn how much your family likes to push you around.). After hearing the most beautiful voice singing a song about the "Gold" and the lighting of the torch, we set out to conquer the Hacienda Business Park sidewalks. Most of the way my dad pushed a wheelchair full of water bottles, but as we pushed on, mom did take a short ride and I did too near the end. We were the very last team to cross this finish line but it felt so good to accomplish something I didn't think I could do. It reminded me of the story I read earlier in the week about a Special Olympics event. As the racers were running down the track, one of them fell. The others took notice, and instead of continuing, all of the racers stopped, walked back to the one who fell, helped him up and all walked hand-in-hand across the finish line, together.

Why do I support the Special Olympics? This event is one of the few great milestones in the life of a person with Developmental Disabilities. While most of us enjoy life's traditional accomplishments (graduation from high school or college, wedding, birth of first child, purchase of first home, etc.) people with DD rarely experience these events. Earning a medal in the Special Olympics is one of the few opportunities to feel that rush of endorphins that come with winning, accomplishing, and fully participating in life.

I plan on continuing to fully participate in life during my cancer gig. This coming Thursday marks the half-way point for my chemotherapy treatments. To quote my dear friend Olivia, "I am too blessed to be stressed." Ask me if I am still quoting her once the construction begins.

Until next week,

Love,

cMc

p.s. I'm not the only one who has a dream. When you share this with others, share with them your dream too.

10/13/02—Cathy Update #21
(14 Weeks Post-Surgery, 4 Days After
4th AC Chemo Treatment)

The Grapes of Wrath

Well, perhaps wrath is a bit strong, how about "The Grapes of Irony." Just before my diagnosis, my friend Dave introduced me to Concannon Winery's Library club, complete with a sneak preview option for being the first to taste their varietal wines before the public. I was so proud to become a lifetime member and receive a magnum of Petite Sirah, my most favorite wine in the world. I have long wanted to become a wine connoisseur and working in a town with wineries, it seems fit that I should know more about wine, considering I like to drink it. Low and behold, I have decided not to make my liver work any harder than necessary during my chemo treatments, and with the exception of my traditional dram of single malt scotch Sunday morning for the Scottish games, I have been alcohol free since my treatments began. This may seem like no big deal, if your liver weren't Irish. I have always walked that fine line, when the doctor's forms ask, "how many drinks per week?? 1-3, 4-6, more than 6? Never knowing where the point of no return is. If my liver is Irish, do I get an extra 2 drinks per week? Is a glass of wine one drink, and a martini worth two? They never give you directions with these types of medical quizzes.

Anyway, I am not one for giving up vices easily (still do the latte, decaf now), especially when my psychological well being is at stake, so I chose to continue drinking wine, in my own way, so that I am not the odd woman out when celebrating with friends and family. Drinking ice tea out of a wine glass can only get you psyched up so much, don't you know. So I am here to share with you my discoveries of alcohol free and de-alcoholized wine, information you may want to know about should you become a designated driver and still want to look the part of a full-blown wine connoisseur.

During my chemo treatment this week (Last AC treatment!! I'm half way done with chemo :-) my mom and I brought some wine to the chemo lounge with cheese and crackers to share. The doctor's got quite a kick out of walking into the treatment room seeing wine glasses at everyone's side table. One doctor, I call him Doctor Bow tie, smiled and said, "I know it isn't wine, I can smell wine a mile away," then he left the room. We were worried he was upset, until we saw him return with a lead crystal champagne flute, arm extended, ready for his share of the beverage. Funny coincidence. Some of the patients remembered that the building we were in used to be a restaurant called the Shannon, and the part of the building that is now the chemo lounge used to be the bar. Some things never change.

During our little happy hour (ok, happy 2.5 hours) mom distributed plastic wine glasses full of Ame beverage and Concannon Grape Juice, our two selections for tasting that day. Ame is made by Orchid Drinks UK and is imported by The Natural Group, Modesto. It has no alcohol and comes carbonated in three flavors (colors) Red, Rose and White. All three flavors have these delicious extracts: schizandra, limeflower, jasmine and gentian. White has 55% grape and 1% Apricot juice. Rose has 55% grape, 2% raspberry and 2% black berry juice. Red has 50% grape, 2% elderberry and 2% lemon juice. They are all very refreshing served chilled. You can find them at Trader Joe's for only $3 a bottle. Our second selection is my favorite non-alcoholic grape juice bottled by Concannon Winery (of course, with my luck, they ran out of this selection and will not have another batch until my chemo treatments are over. This bottle is donated from mom and dad's own private collection). This delicious 1999 vintage juice is a Rhone style combination of 69% Cinsaut, 21% Counnoise, and 10% Grenache noir. Last purchase price was just under $6 per bottle (10% discount for Library club members).

There are other de-alcoholized wines out there, but they do have .5% alcohol by volume. They taste more like wine, as they are wine with most of the alcohol removed. Ariel is a popular brand at around $7 per bottle. I have tasted their Cabernet Sauvingnon, Merlot and Rouge. They also make a Chardonnay which is tasty. They are bottled by Ariel vineyard at the J. Lohr Winery in San Jose. Sutter Home also makes a de-alcoholized wine called Fre ($6). (Fre, Ame, seems three letter names are popular, drop the alcohol, drop the letters). They have Cabernet, Merlot, Chardonnay and White Zinfandel. The Pleasanton Hotel serves Fre White Zinfandel. Having alcohol-free wine is a nice way to feel as if I am participating in my "normal" routine and that I feel I've made one less sacrifice to this cancer gig. It is also a heads up that in the future, when someone else (of course not me) offers to be the designated driver, the least I could do is provide them with a bottle of alcohol free wine to enjoy with dinner. Many restaurants do not carry it, so I plan to bring the bottle myself.

I hadn't had enough during my Happy Hour, I had to go out and party some more that night. Thursday was Tracy's annual Wine Stroll. I pulled out my trusty wheelchair, grabbed a bottle of Red Ame, and hit downtown with a vengeance.

It was nice to get out in the fresh air, and have it be less than 98 degrees. I wasn't planning on attending, considering I had a chemo treatment that day, but I have such good luck with my trusty wheelchair I didn't want to miss out on one of Tracy's major social events. I enjoy the small town atmosphere and running into people I know while strolling the streets (Can't call me a street walker, but maybe a street roller).

Everyday and every week (here she goes again) I still count my blessings for how fortunate I am through all this. Each time I go for a chemo treatment I meet a new patient. This week I met a lovely young woman who is round two with her breast cancer. She was first diagnosed two years ago, when her child was just 2 years old. After 8 months of chemotherapy (4 treatments of AC and Taxol followed by 8 cycles of CMF), she was then diagnosed with ovarian cancer, followed by another breast cancer diagnosis in her opposite breast. She took fertility drugs during her pregnancy and is suspicious that may have stimulated her cancer growth. Another cancer patient sitting in the lounge this week has been receiving treatment here non-stop for 3 years. I have hope that my path doesn't follow suit.

I had a few minor set backs this week that normally would have thrown me for a loop. All in the course of 3 days I discovered that 3 of those closest to me have been laid off of their jobs. My continual struggle to establish DSL services has led me to the forced purchase of a new computer (Hey Dude, we're gettin' a Dell) and the contractor we had lined up for our house remodel has backed out. And guess what!? I didn't cry. I didn't even panic. A part of me realized that these are circumstances that are not mine to control. No amount of worry, concern, crying, etc. would change them. Providing support where it is needed, as I have received in such great abundance, is the most I can provide to my loved ones, that much power I do have. Then I found this prayer while reading in the bath tub last night (Yes, the girl reads prayers in the bath tub. You should try it! Become one with the suds.).

"Protector of All, I care not if all things else are wrested away from me by my self-created destiny; but I shall demand of Thee, mine Own, to guard the slender taper of my love for Thee." As long as I keep the faith, I can handle what comes my way.

Stroll on!

cMc

p.s. Go forth and whine about the wine.

10/21/02—Cathy Update #22
(12 Days After Last AC Chemo Treatment)

Mirror Mirror on the Wall…Oh the Vanity of it All

Being bald for the period of a year can sure have an effect on one's perception of beauty. Men have found solace in the well known belief that being bald is directly related to high testosterone, which in turn, means you are the manliest of men. Women, on the other hand, haven't got a single socially accepted truth to hang out there should we be brave enough to leave home hairless or hatless. We do, however, have the joy of changing headdress on a daily basis should we choose to perceive the gift of baldness as an opportunity instead of a dread. I'm having a blast shocking friends and loved ones with new looks every time they see me. I bought a new wig at Anita's salon last Friday during their sale. Got it half price! I'm now a red head, and as several have stated, just in time for Fall, the color works well this time of year. This new style fits my personality better, as the old wig was too Republican for me and reminded me of Harriet Nelson. It worked well when I was dressed up, but my hippie alter ego with fan sleeves and bell bottoms didn't fit well with the old hair. Watch out! Next week Valley Rags and Wigs in Dublin is having their annual sale. I may be blond by the next time you hear from me.

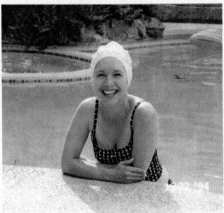

No one knew I had no hair under this cap. Thanks to the placement of Cathy-ter, no one saw an ugly port sticking out from my chest.

As an aside, I want to share with you two jokes from my pal (bald-by-choice) Joe. "If your wig blows off and you chase after it…is that a bald-er-dash?" When on disability for cancer I always have the option to answer the question, "What do you do for a living?" with the response… "I'm bald." Thanks too for the card from Carol this week with a picture of a bald woman, arms full of shampoo, conditioner and products, "What's so great about Chemo?… No Hair. No Hair Care!" Seeing a card made for chemo patients makes me feel "accepted" in a strange way.

I have discovered the ritual of ensembles. Changing hair color brings a whole new variable into coordinating what I wear. I never used to pay attention to assembling a collection of clothing and accessories to coordinate with each other. I used to be more worried about how I looked in my clothes (focusing on the size of my hips and thighs, do I look attractive, and other shallow values) than how the clothes look with each other. Now I catch myself "laying out" a dress and sweater, earrings, necklace, scarf, hat, socks and shoes and changing my selections until I have a symphony of couture in tune with each other. Where does it come from? Why now? I think part of it is developing a camouflaging technique. In order to not draw attention to the head (or lack of hair on it) I want to be seen as a complete unit of style. I would rather be invisible, but I must acknowledge that my job as a sign language interpreter actually calls for people to stare at me for long periods of time. If I can make them comfortable enough to forget I'm bald under that wig or hat, then I have done my job well. Wearing a hat and scarf is not the norm in California, but if I wear an outfit that fits well with it, there will be less tendency for one to perceive the hat as strange.

Besides, I love changing looks from day to day. When I was going to physical therapy weekly (all done now) the therapist's assistant never recognized me from week to week. One week I wore a hat, the next my wig, the next a scarf, the next a different wig. I would plot out how much I could change each week just to throw her off again. My biggest kick out of looking different happened after I cut my hair. I was talking with a friend of mine at the Youth Leadership Forum in Sacramento and I was laughing a lot. When I laugh, my eyes tend to squint, and a long time associate thought I was an Asian visitor to the forum. I've known her for over ten years and she not only didn't recognize me, she profiled me. I fully accepted her compliment as she is Asian herself. Being the sweetheart that she is, she sent me an invitation to a luncheon two weeks ago about Asian women and breast cancer.

It's easier to accept the hair loss knowing there are fun and creative ways to work around the issue and realizing it is a temporary condition. My latest struggle is accepting the lightning speed at which my facial skin is aging. This is permanent and what most women have 10 to 20 years to come to terms with I am facing in the matter of a few months. Chemotherapy can age the skin by 20 years. No matter how much cocoa butter I apply it doesn't seem to slow the process much. I remember watching my mom go through this and noticing years later in pictures that she went from looking younger than her age to looking much older than her age during her cancer experience. I'm worried the same is happening to me. I look in the mirror and notice that in the past two weeks, my chin is starting to look like Tommy Lee Jones (great actor, not very feminine looking chin though). I have been blessed with inheriting Dick Clark genes from my dad and an oily complexion that was my enemy through puberty and my best friend as an adult. One positive side of the chemo is my complexion hasn't looked this clear since my prepubescent years, but that dryness comes with a price. I'm sure all those years of tanning are now slapping me in the face, instead of leaving fingerprints it leaves wrinkles (more like crevasses, canyons even). Normally, you would think, I should be prepared for this since every woman over 40 can expect to start aging, the key term missing here is aging "gracefully" as I am experiencing it with the definition of Divine aging, not slow aging. *(In the long run, my skin didn't age as much as I worried it would)*

My son Paul has inherited a gene from the family, the Portuguese curse. He is the hairiest teenager, with the moniker of "Teenwolf" as an e-mail address. As a teenager this is way cool because he was the first to grow a beard in high school...as a Freshman. His hairy chest intimidates his wrestling opponents to no end. When we went on a train trip to Seattle last year, most people thought he was in is mid-twenties and most people thought I was his girlfriend(smirk). I'm sure my immature behavior was certainly a factor in people's misperception, however I must admit that my complexion up until recently has been fairly wrinkle free, and I am sure my obvious pimple here and there screams youth to an untrained eye. We had the best time on that trip. In first class, they make announcements from the dining car constantly calling out the names of people waiting for their turn, and we gave the name "Osbourne" after our favorite celebrity family. All the college kids thought we were so cool.

I didn't realize how strong an effect that trip had on my ego until this recent cancer experience. I was actually gloating about the experience, for some reason believing that looking young was somehow important. I spend a lot of time reflecting on who I was, how I was, who I am now becoming, and who I want to be. Our society shapes women's minds to believe they must constantly strive to become the media ideal. Billions of dollars are spent on cosmetics, hair dye, diets, fitness programs, surgery and skin care all in hopes that we can preserve our youthful appearance as long as humanly possible. I saw a program last week where two 18 year old girls had liposuction and botox injections and there was NOTHING WRONG with the way they looked. One of the most revealing classes I took while in college (1998) was Sex, Gender and the Arts, an art history course examining the representation of women through out art history and the contributions of female artists. We have been subjected to the "male gaze" since history began (post-apple eating Eve I think) and society has perpetuated women being required to dress, make up and accessorize appropriately to meet the needs of their male audience (except Louis XIV, he was gorgeous). It's so bad that the male audience of critics now includes women so that we not only have to impress men, we must compete to impress other women. That means we are throwing our money at what everyone else wants to see, not what we want for ourselves.

I am worried I am going to look much older when this is through, but how appropriate, I am also going to BE much wiser, so why shouldn't I look the part. I don't need to flaunt my features so I can attract a breeding partner in order to continue my blood lines (which is the only logical explanation for this whole vanity thing in the first place). Perhaps I will gain more respect in the work place as others perceive me to have more experience because "I look the part." I have actually experienced professional sabotage from jealous, insecure middle aged women in the past. I wonder if unattractive women experience the same thing? (Wow, that was a vain statement) Flirting was also common place for me. A young attractive woman wastes so much time being polite yet firm with male suitors. Just think of all the time I will save not having to fend off the masses of deprived men (OK, so maybe I wasn't that popular, it did happen enough to get annoying though). I consider myself lucky. I now have the ideal "excuse" for looking older. Unfortunately, society will excuse me for looking old because I survived cancer as opposed to looking old because "I let myself go" or because "I inherited bad genes." Actually, I would prefer to look older because I didn't give a damn about how society perceived me and I don't play those games and never did. It is hard to change a life-time of brain washing and actually believe this. I'm working on it.

Jamie Lee Curtis was on Oprah the other day (I truly believe God gave me cancer so I could stay home and watch Oprah) talking about her recent children's book about self esteem and her new campaign to combat Hollywood's ongoing beauty contest. She is wearing less make up, giving up the high heel pumps and allowing herself to gain some weight. Most people identify her with the perfect body and yet she is now becoming a spokes person for the very concept I am trying to accept myself...love you for who you are, not what others want you to be. I remember a quote I wrote down from a friend of mine, Edward, "I want to be accepted for who I am, as I am." As someone who has survived a severe brain trauma injury and achieved long term sobriety, he is one of my favorite scholars of life. I've learned so much from him.

So, this old lady hopes to see you soon, though you may not recognize me. I could be a brunette, red head or blond or may be sporting a hat and scarf ensemble, one thing for sure, I'll look sharp. I won't look sharp because I want you to look at me, I'll look sharp because I like to spend the time to coordinate and accessorize so "I" like what I am wearing and it makes ME feel good to wear it.

The hell with the rest of them, I don't appease the "gaze" any more.

Love you,

cMc

p.s. When sharing this with others, don't forget to tell them about the wig sale! You don't have to be bald to join in on the fun!!

10/27/02—Cathy Update #23
(3 days before 1ˢᵗ Taxotere Chemo Treatment)

The Long and Winding Road

(Sing Along: Lyrics by Paul McCartney and John Lennon)

Hearing Paul McCartney sing this song in concert Monday night had special meaning to me. Not only was I hearing a legend and seeing him live on stage, but I was listening to a song that seems to reflect my personal journey, my own long and winding road. My cancer experience has had the most profound impact in my journey to know God and has helped me more than any other event in my life to "let me know the way." I listen to the lyrics of songs now with renewed insight.

Thank you Charlie for my early birthday present (tickets to the concert) and the opportunity to experience the closest thing to a Beatles concert anyone can see today. Thank you to the scientists who have developed chemotherapy treatments to a point that I can still enjoy special moments like this during my treatment.

Paul McCartney is also a survivor. He lost John and George to violence from crazed fans (or anti-fans to be more accurate) and his wife to cancer, yet he has managed to continue to thrive, being knighted by the Queen, and moved on to remarry and start a new life. Humans have an incredible resilience and ability to survive even the most unthinkable challenges. I remember watching an episode of Oprah (here she goes again) where she interviewed a woman who survived the World Trade Center collapse with burns over 80% of her body. She is covered head to toe with tight wraps and undergoes 5 hours every day of physical therapy. She is now back at home with her infant daughter and husband, but has years of therapy to go. I see that and I look at myself and realize my challenges are so small in comparison, how can I feel anything but grateful.

Last week when I said "God gave me cancer so I could stay at home and watch Oprah" I was hinting toward the value and impact this show can have on helping people. I am a huge fan. I have watched several episodes that included topics or speakers that have provided tools for my healing. Just this week she showcased people who have used writing as a tool to heal. Tom DeBaggio writes about his Alzheimers in "Loosing my Mind: An Intimate Look at Life with Alzheimers." A mother and daughter (Kathy and Amy Eldon) published the photos and journals of their son and brother photojournalist Dan Eldon (who died in Samalia) in the book "Angel Catcher: A Journal of Loss and Remembrance." They have also developed several journaling books (Soul Catcher and Love Catcher) to help others begin to write journals to help them with daily life. Michele Weldon writes about how her journal helped her leave an abusive relationship in "Writing to Save your Life: How to Honor your Story Through Journaling."

In a way, these weekly updates are my journal. I write down ideas and little epiphanies that come to me during the week in a journal given to me by a friend early in this process. Even though the pages are falling out and I need to tape them into place, the fact that she gave me this book is symbolic of the many gifts others have given to help me heal. Writing in this particular journal is important to me (especially since the pages are falling out and it appears quite worn). I then review my notes and compose these weekly journals to share with you what is going on in my life, and in my head. Initially I wanted to do this so friends and family knew how I was doing and wouldn't feel compelled to call me and ask. This also gives me more privacy and spending so much time on the phone could be physically draining too. I also wanted to get the details out of the way so when I did talk to someone, we could talk about something other than me and my condition, because they already knew. Eventually I learned the therapeutic powers behind writing. Not only does this process help me heal, as several of you have said, you too gain knowledge and insight from reading what I write. That makes me feel good too. I also figured out another possible outcome of this experience…if one hundred people read my updates each week, that means I am in the minds of one hundred people on a regular basis. I truly believe in the power of prayer and if that many people pray for my recovery on a regular basis, I become the recipient of an incredible healing power (kind of selfish, I realize, but what the hey). The humor I infuse in my writing (although today isn't as funny as usual) not only reflects my twisted sense of humor, but it allows all of us to laugh in the face of cancer. The topic of cancer is so unnerving to people, the ability to find light and laugh "about" (not laugh "at") such a serious topic is empowering. Mind over matter.

My new computer arrived on Wednesday. I now have the tools necessary to consider publishing my updates and join the ranks of other cancer survivors who have found the power of healing in writing. I hope to share with other future cancer patients a weekly diary that can be like a virtual support group, as all of you have been my weekly support group. I also have a new e-mail address to use for personal messages and plan to begin sending my updates from my new address next week. If you have business-related messages please continue to send them to my work e-mail address.

Thank you for being there for me, for writing back and encouraging me to continue my updates. I want you to realize how much you are a part of my healing process.

Until next week,

Write on!

cMc

p. s. Once I start sending updates from my personal e-mail I won't need to write these silly permission slips to share my personal info with others. I'll also be more free to speak my mind on topics inappropriate in the work place. (Oh no, that could be dangerous).

11/3/02—Cathy Update #24
(4 Days After 1st Taxotere Chemo Treatment)

Trick or Treat

My most recent chemo treatment was on Halloween and fortunately it was more treat than trick. I dressed up like a hippy (not really strange for me, but I was more extreme than usual) with a long blond wig, fury psychedelic vest, extreme silver and black eye lashes and purple eye brows. I decorated Cathyter with Halloween tattoos (witch, spider, pumpkin, cat and pitch fork) to give Ses a treat of her own. I handed out lollypops to everyone and proceeded to choke on a piece of mine (since I saved the broken one for me). How ironic would it be for me to choke to death in the chemo lounge from my own candy. I scared poor Ses, so I guess that could be considered a successful Halloween prank (though unintentional). Thanks too Ses for the gift of the book "Uplift: Secrets from the Sisterhood of Breast Cancer Survivors" by Barbara Delinsky. It includes some great tips and hints to help get through treatments.

I don't think people realize the origin of Halloween or understand why we still follow the ritual today. It has been recognized as a Celtic tradition of a fearsome evening where the dead mingled with the living. It is also the eve of All Saints Day where the Catholics considered it a holy celebration of the communion of saints (who happen to be dead too). Trick or treating is only about 40 years old (or so said the web page I got this info from. Others debate with me on this.) and probably started about the time mass production of candy and a healthy economy spawned capitalism to bleed consumers dry for another excuse for a holiday.

What I find most interesting about Halloween is analyzing why adults look forward to the one time each year they have an excuse to dress in costume. For me, it was a chance to have long hair again, thick full lashes, and represent a philosophy of peace in this time of anticipated war. I think most of us take this opportunity to be something we are not, perhaps something we want to be, or something we fear the most about ourselves. Next time you dress in costume, look in the mirror and ask yourself "why did I pick this?"

Is there something missing in your life? Did you dress like a hero? Could you do more to contribute to society? Did you dress like a dancer? Do you secretly want to take tap dancing lessons? Did you dress up sexy? Do you wish something was different in your relationship? We can learn a lot about ourselves from our fantasies. Me, today, I am happy to look in the mirror and say, "I'm breathing! This is good."

My last chemo treatment was my first dose of Taxotere and only took an hour and a half. I took pills the day before, during and after to reduce the side effects of fluid retention. The best part about no longer receiving AC treatments is no more need for anti-nausea medication. That stuff made me loopy for days after each treatment. I do look a little like Gary Coleman ("What you talkin' about Willis?") as my face is a bit swollen, but that should subside soon. Another possible side effect is fluid retention in the lungs and longer periods of anemia, so I need to be extra careful not to catch anyone's cold.

Fuzzy wuzzy is my head. My hair is growing back and a fine spray of gray and brown surrounds my crown like a halo. Some of my old hairs are sticking it out and I scrub to try to move them out of the way so fresh new hair can grow. I don't know if the Taxotere will cause the new hair to fall out or if it will continue to grow. I'm just glad to have a little warmth up there as the nights are getting colder. One new experience that helps to keep me warm are the "private summers" I experience. Each hot flash seems pretty mild and only lasts about 3 minutes, but last week I had at least 20 of these in one day. Glad it's not August.

I have been struggling to get this home computer working with my DSL. I can't believe how incompetent the tech support is with my service provider. All I needed to do was click on one button (and I asked them if I should activate it and they said "no") and once that was checked, all is running smooth now. I couldn't have done it without my friend Gayle. I consider myself somewhat computer literate, but without having a system administrator at home I could spend days trying to figure things out on my own. She is a master with e-mail and home networks, does application installation and tutoring as well as regular maintenance and website design. And she's a sweetheart to boot.

I hope to continue to send my e-mails from my new home e-mail address, barring any unforeseen problems. Please note the return address so we can correspond without going through my work address. It feels nice to now have a space in my home where I sit down, sipping my tea and spend quality time reaching out to friends and family. In the past I have never done much more than an annual New Year letter to update people I know. This morning I replied to cousin Bonnie in Massachusetts and a friend in Hawaii. What a gift this technology is and what a joy to realize the miles melt away when I write to them.

Today I celebrate my 42 birthday. Yesterday while taking a walk I stopped at the swing set in the park and flew through the air for awhile. The air is crisp outside and the leaves are turning.

To quote my favorite Grannie "Ain't life Grand!"

(To be truthful, Grannie used to say "Ain't LOVE grand!" but I think of her any time I hear the word "grand" used in this way)

cMc

11/10/02—Cathy Update #25
(11 Days After 1ˢᵗ Taxotere Chemo Treatment)

Taxotere...Tax of Tears

Initially I was enjoying my new treatment of Taxotere better than AC because I don't have to take those annoying Ativan pills any more. The first several days after treatment were great, then the ugly symptoms began. Many bosom buddies have described to me their symptoms during chemotherapy (sore mouth, feeling in a fog, really tired) and I counted my blessings that I did not experience the same side effects during my AC treatments. I guess my days of skating through chemo are over. I'm having a tough time with Taxotere.

In no way do I want anyone to interpret my description of symptoms as a complaint. I continue to be grateful that what I am experiencing is so much better than the possibility of allowing the cancer to continue to grow. These side effects, as uncomfortable as they may be, are worth the outcome of my treatment. No one said life comes without pain. The worst pain I have experienced in my life was childbirth, and that lead to the most beautiful person in my life, my wonderful son Paul. Well worth it! That's how I see my chemotherapy treatments, and hopefully I can continue that belief to help me through radiation treatments.

So, with that said...I feel like shit! It started about 5 days after my first Taxotere treatment. My ears, throat, lungs and teeth hurt so bad I started taking 600mg of ibuprofen 3 times a day. That helped. Then my tongue developed a thrush-like coating, which went away after a few days, but left my tongue with a terrain similar to Afghanistan *(If I wrote this today, I would say it resembles the landscape of Mars, but I didn't know what Mars looked like then).* My tongue remains sore, with swollen taste buds, and sores are beginning to form on the linings of my cheek. Thanks to the advice of my bosom buddy Betty, I have ordered a mouthwash called "Ulcer Ease" through the local pharmacy. It should arrive Tuesday. That is supposed to ease the mouth pain. Unfortunately, no pharmacy in Tracy or Sacramento carries it, so

I had to order it. Thanks also to another buddy, Susan, for recommending instant mashed potatoes as a chemo patient's best friend. That night when my teeth hurt so bad I couldn't chew, I had that box of potatoes waiting for me in the cupboard. I never tasted anything so good, and so comforting, in my life. 3 minutes to instant bliss.

I'm also experiencing pain in various parts of my arms and chest. The lymph system in my left arm gets shooting (although not severe) pains up and down my arm. I feel pains in my surgery sites too, so I guess the places that are still healing are stimulating my brain to interpret pain. The Taxotere has "neurological" side effects which include numbness and tingling, so what I am experiencing isn't unusual (so they say). I also have episodes when my brain goes into a fog. It's not so bad that it effects my driving, but it is annoying when I make the attempt to think. So, it may be in my best interest not to do any thinking for the rest of my treatments. Who knows what trouble I may get myself into making decisions while "thinking in a fog." I did find solace during one of my walks this week. I went back to that swing in the park. A smile spontaneously broke through my solemn face the second I started to swing. That really perked me up. Cleared up those Taxo-tears.

The worst effect of all that I am experiencing…I'm still full of shit. Literally (do not read the remainder of this section during your lunch hour). I was so constipated that I took double dose laxatives for 5 days, then added stool softeners, until achieving the desired effect. I will now be continuing the stool softeners for the remainder of my chemo treatments. While awaiting the "desired effect" I lived my life on the edge, never knowing when the "movement" was going to happen, or how much time I would have to get to a bathroom. I was scared to drive long distances, or make any time commitment, longer than 10 minutes at a time. I realized how precarious it was for me to accept a one-hour interpreting assignment (in front of an audience of 100) right after having a full body massage during my lunch break (What if the massage "shakes something loose?"). I visualized myself running up the aisle half way through the meeting, hoping the restroom was within sprinting distance. Then God stepped in and cancelled my interpreting assignment. Whew! Then, to remind me of his twisted sense of humor, my massage appointment cancelled too. Oh well, that left only one concern, will I make it on the drive home without having a blow out? And I'm not talking about my tires. Never before have I contemplated what it must be like, what a prisoner one would be, to live under constant fear of "leakage." To be dependent on Depends. I have a new found sensitivity for that population.

Driving this week had two profound impacts on me. Surviving on the road during my "urgency" condition was one thing, surviving the first rainfall of the season was another (People don't slow down...duh!). I was more afraid to drive on the freeway during the first rain than I am of getting cancer again (Californians don't know how to drive in the rain). Dying in a car accident, or any instant cause of death, has the opposite affect of the cancer experience. It is instant, no time for goodbye. You have seconds for your life to pass in front of you before it's gone. Cancer, on the other hand, at least buys you some time. For some it buys them months, for others who catch it early it buys them an entire new life. I have time to tell my loved ones how much they mean to me, and I have. I have time to reflect on my past, forgive myself for my mistakes, accept myself for my imperfections, and move forward with a renewed perception of who I am. Despite what I am going through, no BECAUSE of what I am going through, I have never been happier. I now have the ability to live the rest of my days (and hopefully there will be at least 19,000 more) aware of how precious life is, appreciating each day as a gift, and living accordingly. I call this my "cancer induced awakening." It's a shame it took cancer for me to snap out of it (or into it). My hope is that these weekly updates will not only benefit other bosom buddies, but will have some impact on the rest of you to realize you too have time to change. Don't wait for cancer to affect you. If you too drive on the freeway during the first rain of the season, you may not have tomorrow. What better day than today to begin living. Truly living.

"If only I did___" doesn't exist in my vocabulary.

Stay dry!

cMc

p.s. Wedding date is set. August 10, 2003. Ain't Love Grand!

11/17/02—Cathy Update #26
(3 days before 2nd Taxotere Chemo Treatment)

Mowf Pobems

'iss week my mowf hurt besuz I have ussers fum my yass sheemo heameh. Oh, that's right, I can type clearly, I don't have to type like I sound. Interpretation: "This week my mouth hurts because I have ulcers from my last chemo treatment." At one point I envisioned a troupe of 200 pound, 6 foot tall transvestites in Beach Blanket Babylon attire doing the Riverdance on my tongue, wearing stiletto heels. I feel much better today. Actually, today my tongue has improved so much I can go without medicating it all day and I haven't needed any ibuprofen yet today. That Taxotere really has been a struggle. I have ulcers in the back of my throat, and on the tip of and underneath my tongue. These made talking and swallowing painful, not to mention the precariousness of eating and the excruciating pain of toothpaste.

I have had some wonderful advice from friends for remedies for ulcers. Ulcer Ease is a mouthwash with phenol, an oral anesthetic, yet Chloroseptic actually has a higher does of phenol in it. These provided brief relief. Another suggestion which helped is to suck on Tums to reduce the acid in the mouth and sooth the sores. My bosom buddy Ann and I met for tea and latte this week (I admire this woman so much. She was stage III, double mastectomy and two weeks after surgery she flew to Alaska to see her new baby granddaughter. She is a special education teacher and only misses school on the day she has her chemo treatment. Wow!). She is exactly one week ahead of me in her treatments although she is receiving Taxol instead of Taxotere. I gave her the list of ingredients for my oncologist's Magic Mouth rinse (equal parts Lidocaine 2%, Nystatin and Maalox, swish and swallow). This actually tastes pretty awful, but it did numb my mouth for up to 15 minutes. I would rinse my mouth with this before meals and before brushing my teeth. When it got really bad, I would apply the Lidocaine with a Qtip directly to the sore spots. Unfortunately I can't reach the sores in the back of my throat. Once the ulcers came to the surface I applied Zilactin canker sore medicine (benzocaine) to the sores. This hurts like H-E-double toothpicks because it has alcohol in it, but once it dries it leaves a protective coating over the sore that relieves the pain for many hours. Keep your fingers crossed that I don't get these again after my next treatment. With the AC, my symptoms subsided as my body adjusted to the treatments and hopefully the same will happen with the Taxotere.

I had a reunion with Papa Smurf on Tuesday, my 3-month post surgery follow up. He wasn't wearing his bright blue scrubs, but he was considerate enough to wear a blue shirt to stay in tune with his Smurf theme. I just love that guy. He is warm and funny, compassionate and reassuring (I'm not just saying that because he reads my updates). After examining me he said I was "perfect," a standard I refuse to aspire to. I told him I am accustomed to being "good enough for government work" but he assured me I am doing better than that. He did an ultrasound of the cyst in my right breast (I have had for almost 2 years now). It still looks, feels and behaves like a cyst so I'm not going to worry my pretty little head over that for now (*It has since disappeared*). We discussed my weight gain. I have gained 10 pounds (the average for a breast cancer patient on chemo) and refuse to reduce my calorie intake at this time of my life. I thought perhaps my mouth ulcers are God's way of telling me to stop eating so much. The weight gain is caused by a combination of chemo medications, lack of exercise (hello, I'm too tired to workout for an hour every day), birthday cakes (my sister-in-law made me two…oh so good) and Halloween candy. Papa Smurf reminded me of the positive side to gaining weight while on chemo, "it's a good sign that you aren't dying." I like that perspective.

During my weekly check up with Dr. Bangladesh he informed me that my blood counts are extremely low. My white blood cell counts during AC were within the low end of the normal range most of the time (around 4), but during Taxotere I have dropped to 2 during one week and .9 during the other (sorry, can't recall which week was worse). It's strange that I don't feel that tired and the fog I had the first week wasn't there this past week. My main concern with having such low counts is catching a cold or the flu. I already missed seeing my brother for my birthday because he had a cold and didn't want to infect me. Now I'm going to miss seeing my niece for a family get together this week because she has been exposed to the Coxsackie Virus at pre-school (sounds like something Linda Lovelace would catch, not my sweet innocent 3 year old niece). One of my co-workers came to work sick two weeks ago and infected at least 3 of us. Too-blessed-to-be-stressed Olivia gave her a tongue lashing for coming to work with a fever. I caught a sore throat from her and had a slight fever for about 4 days, but thank heaven that is gone and I seemed to be able to fight it off. The sore throat remains though, and I'm not sure if it is from an ulcer or is residue from that cold, or perhaps I already have the Coxsackie virus (which includes symptoms of sores in the back of the throat). My other co-workers are trying to convince me to wear a face mask while at work, but I can't seem to bring myself to doing that (Visions of Howard Hughes and Michael Jackson perhaps getting in the way). I did scrub my desk, keyboards mouse and telephone at work this week to reduce the germs there (Yuck. When was the last time you cleaned yours? I thought I was a clean person until I finished that nasty chore).

The highlight of my week was a trip to Mill Valley and Sausalito this weekend. My friend David invited friends to hear his new comedy material and get feedback on his latest routines. Before hearing David's schtick, Charlie and I visited with him while strolling through downtown Mill Valley. We then strolled through Sausalito and had dinner with a view of San Francisco city lights across the bay. I love watching the moonlight dance on the surface of the ocean and bay waters. It sparkles like diamonds against the black velvet waves. A nice romantic evening, with a soft vegetable polenta meal (Taxotere forces me to focus on food's texture instead of taste).

David is a humorist and motivational speaker. I mentioned him in an earlier update when he was the key note speaker at the Youth Leadership Forum for disabled high school students last summer. David has a "facial difference" ('disfigured' or 'deformed' are considered too harsh to use in this day and age of political correctness) yet he has dreamy eyes and a warm inviting voice which delivers his quick wit and sense of humor. David has been performing his "Church of 80% Sincerity" routine for years in which he transforms from a person with a facial difference to a beautiful person by the end of the routine. It is a transformation that compels the audience to see themselves in him as they learn about his life story and his perception of how society treats people who are different. He does all this while you roll in the aisle laughing. It's quite a trick. His new material invites you to challenge your perception of what God is like and he throws in some hilarious material about reaching middle age and how people with disabilities are going to take over the world. It's great stuff. I encourage you to see him perform if you can. Visit his website at DavidRoche.com.

David is one of the reasons why I am handling my cancer experience so well. It is through friendships with people with disabilities that I have learned that everyone has the ability to take life's curve balls and hit a home run. What I am currently experiencing is so minor compared to the daily challenges, DAILY challenges, that some people with disabilities endure for their entire life time. How can I be anything but grateful that my symptoms are temporary and I will return to being quote unquote normal. I know many people with disabilities don't like to be labeled "heroes" because that singles them out as super human or some how not the norm when they are just normal human beings. Many don't like being called "inspirational" because they are just living their lives as best they can and they don't ask to be a role model for anyone. Perhaps the reason they reject these acknowledgements is because it brings them attention, and people have been staring at people with disabilities forever, and many want to live their life without being the center of attention. Anonymity is a precious gift only the "normal" can enjoy. In my opinion, my friends and acquaintances with disabilities are my heroes. Firefighters and police officers have been famous as heroes for risking their lives for others, yet they made a choice to do that. People with disabilities did not choose to become disabled, yet they endure society's barriers to lead ordinary, and for some extraordinary, lives.

Thank you David, and all my other dear friends, for without you I would not have developed the ability to endure this experience with such comfort and Grace.

Love,

cMc

11/25/02—Cathy Update #27
(5 days after 2nd Taxotere Chemo Treatment)

Ob-La-Di, Ob-La-Da, Life Goes on, Bra…La, La How Their Life Goes on.
(Sing Along: Lyrics by Paul McCartney and John Lennon)

In the midst of my experience I realize that life goes on, milestones pass, plans for the future continue despite what I am going through. My mouth found happiness again as my ulcers healed. Work was really busy last week. The holidays are just ahead. Hey, this sounds like I still have a life.

My "baby" turned 18 last Monday. This milestone brings both happiness and sorrow. He's a fine young man and I am so proud. The thing that keeps me from crying is his decision to live at home while going to college (yipee). What struck me the hardest was when he filled out the forms for the "Selective Service." How precious we hold life in times of illness and war. Why not everyday? Why not treasure our child because today they are turning 5 years and 45 days old?

Another milestone we celebrated this week included a trip back down to Encinitas (not Encinada) for our friend Henry's 50th birthday. I felt well enough to travel and fortunately my mouth remained functional long enough to enjoy the French cuisine and Katie's exquisite rum cake (the last thing I tasted before my mouth 'turned' on me again was that yummy cake).

Plans for the future also continue as we shopped for motels while down south. We found accommodations for our families close to the beach where we will marry next summer. We also opened our first joint bank account together (hey, check out Tracy Federal Bank's 3.25% CD rate with new checking account). *(Depending on what year you read this, that rate may seem outrageous)*. Then this morning our architect called with questions about the window measurements for the remodel project. Geez, all this planning sure sounds like someone expects to have a "happily ever after."

My last chemo treatment was up in the air as my red blood cell counts were still fairly low. Fortunately my white counts went up (thanks to that cold) and the doctor felt it was safe to go ahead with treatment. I've been eating broccoli and spinach like crazy to bring my counts up again. Spinach is the easiest quick veggie fix, just get a bag of pre-washed spinach and eat it straight from the bag or heat for one minute in a bowl in the microwave. I also found the greatest way to prepare broccoli that's quick and easy, tastes great and has extra protein.

Melt 1/2 stick margarine with 1/2 cup pine nuts and 1/3 cup raisins in saucepan. Add 2 tablespoons lemon juice and pour over steamed broccoli. Yummmm!

My energy level is really, really low these past few days. Henry's wife Joni suggested I try Gatorade or any drink with electrolytes. Joni has a friend whose energy was revived during her chemo treatments by drinking electrolytes. It's certainly worth a try. I'm sipping away right now.

I've also been super paranoid this week because Charlie came down with a cold. I suspect I gave it to him since I was fighting one myself, but I couldn't be sure. I didn't know if I could get sick from him or not so I took no chances. Poor man. I've been merciless. As we traveled together in the car I wouldn't let him touch the radio dials. Every time he touched something I would remind him that he was "infecting us all." I asked him to wash his hands first before he reached for a door knob or picked up something. I watched him like a hawk, anticipating his next move, ready to pounce with an "a-a-a don't touch that." I slept in another room and refused to use the same bathroom he used. Where are those quarantine suits when you need one? Poor Charlie felt like a character in the movie "Outbreak," and I was the Director (sorry Honey! Survival instincts totally took over). It is a quandary though. What do you do when someone you live with gets sick? Fortunately for Charlie, he gets a reprieve by going home today after dropping me off in Tracy. But he had 4 days of hell living in small quarters with paranoid low-count Lulu (that would be me) glaring at him from across the room.

I am getting a bit weary, and although I have only brief bouts of misery, I continue to try and keep a "stiff upper lip" through all this. By the way, who the heck invented that saying? What does a stiff upper lip look like? Does it stick out straight like a duck's bill? Is it pulled in tight against the teeth? Is there a picture of someone sporting one in National Geographic somewhere? Let me know if you find out. I'd love to share that one.

As I face this coming week, anticipating those painful ulcers, realizing I won't be able to taste Thanksgiving, I once again count my blessings. I don't need to gain any more weight and the holiday meals haven't even started yet. My mouth remedies will help keep my pain level down and neutralize any flavor. If I can't taste anything, I might as well eat all vegetables. Why waste the sweets. I call it "Chemo Cathy's Guide to Holiday Weight Loss." A numb mouth is the way to a flattering figure. Taxotere, Dexetrim, they all sound the same to me.

So this Thursday is Thanksgiving. This is going to be a special one for me. I dare all of us to look at our loved ones across the table this year and say openly just how thankful we are for what we have…for WHO we have in our lives. If we do this I anticipate two types of reactions. 1. Everyone will glow from the revelations and leave feeling inspired to appreciate the holiday season to come or… 2. You will become a blubbering, emotional being who needs to be carried to the couch closest to the Kleenex box. I aspire to be the former, yet expect to become the latter.

Happy Thanksgiving everyone! I am thankful for having you as an essential part of my recovery.

Love,

cMc

12/01/02—Cathy Update #28
(11 Days After 2nd Taxotere Chemo Treatment)

Gobble, Gobble

Thanksgiving truly was a blessing. I did NOT develop mouth ulcers as I did with my first Taxotere treatment, therefore I was able to eat anything I wanted during the long holiday weekend. Although I couldn't taste much (taste buds still whacked) everything felt good, especially the Courvoisier (French brandy) I sipped after Thanksgiving dinner.

These past 3 days were about family and friends for me. Thanksgiving dinner was spent at our friend John's house. Traditional turkey dinner in the company of friends, drinking from Grandma's finest crystal, fire burning in the fireplace, chemistry experiment on the stove top hoping to become a clump free gravy, football game on TV, Maggie the dog chasing moles in the backyard (dug a hole so wide she can fit her head in it), topped off with a friendly (although cut throat) game of Monopoly. As predicted, when we went around the table talking about what we are thankful for, it took all my strength to say the simplest statement, "I'm glad to be alive" before breaking down in tears. You see, I am not nearly as eloquent verbally as I am in writing. Perhaps that is why I go on for so long in these updates. What comes out of the fingertips is far more pleasing, and amusing, than my common vernacular.

Friday morning we drove to San Leandro to have breakfast with our friends Bobbe and Jim and their daughter visiting from college, Tovah. We haven't seen each other in over a year. I want to be more cognizant of these long gaps of time and become more vigilant scheduling time to visit dear friends more than once each year. That morning I realized how much I miss spending time visiting friends.

Later that day we visited one of my best friends (Ruthy) who is up from L.A. for the holidays. We lit the menorah candles and exchanged gifts on the first night of Hanukah. I now have the most fabulous faux fur hat to wear on these cold evenings. I was the stylish Russian looking woman in the Chinese restaurant that evening. Her sister found a red wig in a garage sale earlier in the week (worth at least $300 and in great shape). After I tried it on we put it on her dad Sid. I can't wait until that photo gets developed. I need to add it to my Wig gallery collection, it was priceless. After dinner we went to Temple and during the service, people called out the names of people to pray for who are ill. When Ruthy's mom called out my name, I lost it again (Just can't figure out why I am so teary these days). Ruthy and I held hands. When was the last time you held hands with another adult? (not your significant other). When we were children, it was OK, but for some reason as adults we don't share the same public displays of affection. Holding her hand was such an incredible symbol of our love for each other, regardless of what others think. That was a moment of Grace I'll never forget. Thanks for being such a wonderful friend Ruthy.

The Saturday after Thanksgiving is our annual family reunion. One of the things I love about my family is they appreciate each other enough to have two reunions each year. The Portuguese Picnic is held the last Saturday of June and the Scottish side of the family has a reunion that bounces back and forth between Fresno area and San Francisco Bay Area. I was petrified of catching someone's germs as we now have many children running around with colds. When we arrived I parked myself at a table in the corner so I could see everyone clearly yet have the table as a barrier to prevent children from running up and hugging me (I felt bad being so distant because I adore children, but this was a survival technique that allowed me to comfortably enjoy the day without paranoia taking hold). What a joy to sit back and observe multiple generations of my family all together. Just this past week we lost Uncle Gil (my grandfather's brother, aged 90). He was the last of his generation in our family. Now I watch my cousin's grandchildren running around the house. My son Paul becomes a favorite cousin to the middle children (ages 8-10) as they enjoy climbing on him and beating him up (it's a boy thing, I guess). Jenny's baby boy is the youngest (18 months), yet there is another bun in her oven for us to enjoy at the next reunion. Family! Another blessing to cherish on my journey.

Many of you responded to my last e-mail. I just love it when I hear from you. Remember my friend Joan who gave me the cross blessed by the Pope? Remember her incredible story about Rome that I shared during a past update? (I am breaking my own rule here by starting these sentences with the word "remember." I have had such a bad time with my memory during Chemo treatments I have banned the word "remember" from our household).

Anyway, Joan sent me the most eloquent reply telling me what she is thankful for this Thanksgiving. I MUST share her with you once again for she has found a way to express appreciation for life in a manner that is pure poetry.

From Joan:

"Never being the type to pass up a good game of Truth or Dare, I accept your challenge, and will hopefully have the courage to voice my thoughts while the turkey is being served...

I'm thankful for waking up this morning, and for every other morning that I smacked the alarm off with a moan and a grumble, taking for granted the gift of each new day.

I'm thankful for the ability to function once I manage to get up, every mundane task being a complex series of motor skills that I never once stop to think about or be grateful for achieving.

I'm thankful I have a decent mortgage, a house full of pets, a yard full of weeds, a well-stocked refrigerator, a car that's paid for, too many clothes in the closet, and an office with nice carpet and a big window so I can look out and see the trees and the sun and the rain and smile.

I'm thankful for my friends. Is that a cliché, or what? I'd like to thank my producer, my director... I don't have many friends, never have; I'm a hard person to get close to. Here's to the brutally honest people I can dump on, call in sheer panic, yak at, and feel comfortable with telling my innermost personal stuff. You have my deepest sympathy!

I'm thankful for my family. There's nothing quite like the paradox of witnessing your mother regress as your daughter matures. It's painful, blackly comical, ironic, and produces intense reactions that encompass the emotional spectrum. But I wouldn't miss it for the world.

My mom drives me nuts sometimes; it's hard living with your mother under the best of circumstances, let alone when she's 86 and homebound and frail and forgetful and lonely. I'm thankful to have had her in my life for so long, and will continue to be there to care for her—as she did me.

I'm thankful my dad lived long enough to know his granddaughter, to share songs, movies, and bowls of popcorn;

thankful for the memories of his smile when Amanda cart wheeled up and down the nursing home hall.

Amanda—my joy, my most perfect achievement, my cause for occasional bouts of temporary insanity—my life. As I watch my daughter grow into a young woman, my head swims with shadows of the young girl who was me, and the heartache she caused herself and those who loved her. The effects of a somewhat twisted life have hardened me. I hadn't planned to turn into a cynical old bitch—when did THAT happen? I could jump on the bandwagon and blame my parents, my upbringing, the fact that I was confined to a playpen without food or drink for days and weeks on end (I'm thankful for my endless ability to weave a good yarn), but of course I'd know better. Suffice it to say that I screwed up numerous times over the years, and can't point the finger. Yet my feelings for this child, this soon-to-be-woman, this incredible human being that I somehow miraculously produced, has helped me understand that I really am capable of loving another person. I would fight for her. I would kill for her. I would die for her. And for that I am thankful.

And if I can manage to say all this without slobbering into the mashed potatoes, I'll be truly thankful."

Thank you Joan!

Until the next update.

Thankfully yours,

cMc

12/9/02—Cathy Update #29
(2 Days Before 3rd Taxotere Chemo Treatment)

It's the Pits

These past few days I feel almost normal (normal to me may be a bit skewed compared to most). My energy level is good, my mouth feels fine. I feel pretty darn good for Chemo Cathy.

Last week when I was feeling really tired I remembered someone loaned me a necklace a few months ago to help me heal. It has 3 stones in it, one clear stone with a slightly pink hue, one purple and white stone with a whirly pattern and one green stone. Since I started wearing this necklace last week (24/7, only take it off to bathe) I feel great. Now, I don't completely understand the power of crystals and stones. I am trying to learn more. There could be metaphysical powers at work here or it may simply be my own psychosomatic powers helping me feel better. Either way, if it works, I'm there. So if someone offers you an object that has the powers to help you heal, please give it a try. As long as it doesn't replace your medical procedures to help cure your ailments, what's the harm. I'll accept anything that helps me heal.

The girl's got hair!! I can't believe my hair has already begun to grow back, and I still have two more chemo treatments to go. I show it to everyone I can, pulling back my wig and exposing my butch to everyone's delight. The funniest part is when they see my TRUE hair color, I hear all kinds of questions. "Was your hair that gray before?" being the most common. I dyed my hair for years before it fell out so no one knew what my true color is. My mom calls me "salt and pepper." Paul just calls me "old." At our family reunion I looked at my two aunt's hair color and realized I have more gray than they do. My hair began to turn gray during my 6 year stint of going to college while working full time. That stress level is enough to turn any single parent gray. I'm just grateful my hair didn't fall out while in college (I sure felt like pulling my hair out at times).

I also celebrated another important milestone in my healing process this week. I shaved my arm pits!! Why celebrate? 'Cuz my pits are hairy enough to need shaving, that's why. Hair on my head, hair in my pits. Life is Grand! I think this should become a ritual for all female chemo patients, like something you read about in National Geographic. "The ChemoCat tribe celebrates her emergence into womanhood with the armpit shaving ceremony attended by all other women in the tribe." I could start a new tradition (Flashback: I remember when I was a little girl, I would call my mom's underarm hair her "beard" because my dad had a beard. You know how kids think. I somehow labeled all large quantities of body hair as beards). I have also labeled the hairy characteristics in my family as "the Portuguese curse" not realizing that this curse would become a blessing for a chemo patient. Thanks to the genetic strength and natural abundance of our hair, I didn't have to bear the emotional trauma of living without eyebrows and eyelashes. My brows and lashes remained plenty thick (I remember how worried I was that I would lose my eyebrows and eye lashes). When I was 5 years old, my friend's mother shaved her eyebrows and drew in this heavy brown mass instead. Gave me nightmares. She looked like Joan Crawford. I prayed that I wouldn't look like her through chemo). I never completely lost all the hair on my head and I've needed to shave my legs through this whole ordeal (I say needed, but notice I didn't say that I actually shaved them). While I enjoyed not having to shave under my arms during chemo, the return of my hair makes me feel even closer to this whole ordeal being over with.

Not much else to report this week. My next chemo treatment is this coming Thursday. My last treatment is January 2. Keep thinking about me because your thoughts and prayers sure seem to be helping.

For those of you who know Cupcake (Michael), his surgery is scheduled for Thursday December 12 at San Ramon Medical Center. Please pray extra hard for him that day. He will be there for at least 5 days and visitors are welcome.

Good luck with your holiday shopping!! Until we read again,

bye for now,

cMc

12/15/02—Cathy Update #30
(4 days after 3rd Taxotere Chemo Treatment)

What Goes Up, Must Come Down...the Cancer Roller Coaster Ride

Why do we knock on wood when we say something we are afraid will back fire? Should have done that during my last update. No sooner had I boasted about my healthy head of hair than it began to fall out again. I was getting attached to that black and gray pattern (especially the two gray patches right where my horns once grew) and people were always asking to pet my head. Short lived adventure. It's not as hard emotionally to lose my hair the second time around. At least I know how fast it will grow back. Keep those fingers crossed that the eyelashes and brows remain defiant.

This experience, however, is trivial compared to what faces my dear friend Michael. I went to visit Cupcake in the hospital on Friday (I was actually able to find a plant at Safeway that had a toy cupcake as part of the decoration...amazing). Michael and I were going to battle our cancers together and we looked forward to the future when we would look back and remember how this experience bonded us as friends. He was supposed to have his colon removed on Thursday to rid him of his cancer. They couldn't operate. The cancer has anchored itself to his bones and the chemo and radiation treatment he has already suffered through didn't do enough to make it operable. I was there when the social worker discussed hospice options with him. His determination to fight is incredible. He hasn't thrown in the towel yet. He wants to try a more aggressive chemo treatment before giving up. He still has such a strong attitude of hope and faith. I have learned so much from him these past few months.

There, But for the Grace of God, Go I

I cried all the way home, in the rain. Seems the heavens are also crying for him this weekend.

That night I filled the house with candle light and a fire in the fireplace while listening to Nat and Natalie Cole's Christmas carols. Sherri, Paul's girlfriend, surprised me by decorating the house with seasonal cheer, garlands and lights several weeks ago. I plugged in all the lights. Michael told me how much he enjoys looking at Christmas lights. I grabbed Charlie by the hand and we slowly danced by the glow of the fire.

I am truly blessed. Sheryl Crow is right... it's not having what you want, it's wanting what you have.

Pray for Michael. Pray for a miracle. It's the season for miracles!!

cMc

12/22/02—Cathy Update #31
(11 Days After 3rd Taxotere Chemo Treatment)

Traditions

As you have learned by reading my many, many, many updates, I love my annual traditions. July 4th block party, Scottish Games, wine strolls, walk-a-thons, family reunions, to name a few. One of my favorite annual traditions is Girl's Day at Union Square.

I can't remember when we started going to Neiman Marcus in San Francisco with my great aunt Clara for lunch during the holiday season. I think it's been almost 20 years. I was shocked to read an article in Reader's Digest (or was it TV guide?) that described our tradition as a common one for many San Franciscan women (I wanted to be unique). After nibbling on popovers and lunching at the Rotunda restaurant overlooking Union Square, we leisurely stroll through the store (aunt Clara always stopped to try on fur coats and picked up fruit cake (ew) at the confection counter) before heading out to the square. In the good old days, Gumps had puppies and kittens from the shelter displayed in elaborately decorated window abodes awaiting adoption. We would stroll through Tiffany's and Saks Fifth Avenue, drooling. A stop at the St. Francis to use the restroom was always a treat. These days, the ritual has changed a bit. Clara has since passed, but with the little inheritance she left my parents, she is now paying for our lunch and the limo ride from Fremont to S.F. and back. My mom and I now bring my sister-in-laws and nieces with us (at the ages of 3 and 4, the limo is a must) and instead of Tiffany's and Saks, we now head straight for the Disney Store after lunch.

But This Year I Couldn't go. I Got the Stomach Flu!

Now before you start to feel sorry for me, let me explain how God works in mysterious ways. I can always enjoy this annual tradition for years to come, but if not for the flu, I would have missed the following few days at home, staying with my parents...and I would have gained even more weight eating at holiday parties that week.

There's No Place Like Home. There's No Place Like Home

Since the drive back to Tracy was so far, and the weather was terrible, I decided to stay at my parent's home and let mommy take care of me for three days of bliss (Well, OK, throwing up ain't bliss, but throwing up in the comfort and surroundings of Mom and Dad is a whole lot better than being alone). I didn't grow up in this house, only lived there for about 3 years, but it is filled with all the memorabilia of my childhood and the love of my parents…it feels so safe. Soaking in my old bathtub, sipping 7-up, eating Jello and saltines, staring at the old white porcelain barf pan I grew up with; takes me back to childhood days. I think this feeling I experienced is why it feels so good for us to go "home" for the holidays, to be surrounded by familiar furniture and objects; the bright orange macramé hanging I made in junior high (egad that thing is tacky), the napkin holder my brother made in wood shop, the sauce pan with no handle (broke over 30 years ago), our senior pictures still sit on the mantle in the family room. And there is nothing quite like the smell of mom's baking this time of year, unless, of course, you consider eating the end result.

I drove back home to Tracy on Wednesday during the break between storms and continued to convalesce there, drinking Ensure and lying around like a sack of potatoes. After a few days I called Michael to find he was home from the hospital. I felt a sudden surge of energy and motivation to get out of bed and visit him to see if there is anything I can do to help. After 5 days of feeling drained and self-absorbed I realized, hey, it could have been so much worse. I could have felt like this the entire time I was on chemo. This is as bad as I'm going to feel. It's all up hill from here (Or is it down hill? Idioms confuse me). I only have one more treatment to go. There is light at the end of the tunnel. This was the turning point from feeling as if I was going through chemo treatments to feeling like I am coming out of treatments. This thought was spurred by changing my perspective from looking at me to looking outward to help a friend in need. Thank you Michael for this gift. The joy I lost during my flu episode has returned. I was at the store as soon as it opened and I bought fleece apparel and a blanket to help keep Michael warm, a gift to him from me and my generous gang at work. Giving feels so good!

This is a season for joy. I received a beautiful e-mail reply from a very special bosom buddy this week. She is a friend of my mom's, our neighbor from 37 years ago, Phyllis. She shared with me this sentiment about joy:

"As a 17 year breast cancer survivor, your updates have jolted me into a reality I had lost. When I was going through my experience, I truly felt how lucky I was and my eyes were opened to the wonders of life. After a few years, I still appreciated the wonders of God, but not with the intensity and joy I had following my treatments. You have made me so aware of those wonderful feelings again. Thank you for making me look through your eyes to again feel that wonder and appreciation, an appreciation of life, of family and dear friends. Thank you for your gift."

I was at my mom's house when I read this message out loud to her. We cried and embraced in the joy that we are a sisterhood of survivors.

This Is Why I Write

What I love about this holiday season is that, if only for a fleeting moment, enormous numbers of people feel joy again. It's in the air. It's a season when we shift our priorities to realign with what is really important: family first, gifts and charity, spread joy, have hope, feel peace (not just between countries, but also between the ears).

I look forward to more annual traditions this coming week. Christmas Eve dinner with my friend Fugly's family (I'm their adopted daughter, so to speak) in Modesto and Christmas day in Fremont with my family (Charlie's family is in New Jersey, sigh). We must be home by 5:30 Christmas day so Charlie can participate in one of his favorite traditions… the Kings and Lakers game.

From Me and Mine

To You and Yours,

Have a Joyous and Peaceful Holiday Season!

cMc

12/29/02—Cathy Update #32
(4 days before 4th Taxotere Treatment, Last Chemo)

Ode to a Dad

Four days and counting until my last chemo treatment. Timing couldn't be better. January 2, 2003 is the beginning of a new year, a new life. As these past 6 months drag on, my fatigue weighs more and more. I can't wait to have energy again, to experience the endorphin rush of an hour-long exercise regime, to sweat from physical exertion. I can't wait to exercise discipline over my eating, counting the points (points = weight watchers) to ensure weight loss and health. Have you ever heard of someone wanting these things? I'm sure my bosom buddies can relate. I can't wait, I can't wait.

Both Mom and Dad have been sick with sinus colds since last week so we postponed our Christmas celebration until New Years day (yes, we are a blend of Judaism and Christianity, and like many other capitalists, we celebrate both holidays). I've been thinking a lot about my family during these holidays, especially after spending time at home with my parents during my stomach flu episode. I especially enjoyed spending time with my Dad. I've spoken often of my Mom during my updates (that's Saint Missy to you) but I haven't said much about Dad.

This Update Is Devoted to My Dad

I can only imagine how he felt when he found out about my cancer. He went through this with his wife 17 years ago, and now his little girl. He is silent in his pain, not sharing his sense of helplessness. He has always been able to fix just about anything. Although he is not actively participating in my treatment, as my Mom is, he is always on the other end of the phone when ever I need him.

I'm Daddy's little girl. Ever since he retired I've noticed that he drops what ever he is doing when I come over and gives me his undivided attention. When I was growing up he traveled often and worked incredibly hard (it's a family trait) so he didn't spend as much time with me as a modern day Dad would, yet I have fond memories of him coming to my rescue when ever I was in need. Visions of him running in slow motion toward me fill my memories. When I rode my bike down the hill and crashed into our neighbor's garage door, there he was, running in slow mo (The emergency room had a bed with my name on it. I was a bit of a tom boy, and accident prone). When I fell off the fence and had the wind knocked out of me (same year), there he was, running in slow mo toward me, only this time I was stuck watching the football game with him and Mr. Barnum, eating bugles off my fingertips (remember those?) until I felt better. Even as an adult, when my 3 year old son Paul had a run in with a plate glass window, Dad held me in the emergency waiting room while Paul received 3 layers of stitches in his face. He has always been there for me when I need him.

I reflect on his qualities and feel pride:
Practical, ethical, moral, frugal and all those other–als;
High integrity, honesty, a strong work ethic;
Humorous, witty, sarcastic, intelligent;
Analytical, ingenious, inventive, engineering;
Talented (piano, ukulele, singing, dance, pilot, Mr. fixer-upper);
Cookie Monster!!
Just to name a few.

His nickname for me is Sis, I guess because I am the only girl and sister to two. He was firm with me when I stepped out of line (I didn't expect a spanking when I ran away from home, but in retrospect, I needed it. I did it because I was bored.). He never expected me to live up to anything I couldn't do. He set examples for us to live by, and darn it, he was always right (most of the time). An example of the fine man he is was very evident to our family when it came time for him to give up flying. My Dad dreamed of being a pilot his whole life, yet he only enjoyed the privilege of flying for about 10 years. Instead of allowing a male ego to dictate his life, when he realized that he was forgetting certain steps in his pre-flight checks, he realized that the consequences of those mistakes could be fatal. High blood pressure also lurked in the background. He swallowed his pride, and his dream, and sold his plane (named Tweety Bird) before anything bad could happen.

I wrote my Dad this poem when he sold his plane years ago.

Ode to Tweety Bird

When you were just a wee Lad
You gazed fondly toward the sky
And every day you dreamed about
How some day you would fly

College and Navy, Missy and kids
Your duty to others came first
Then came the day you owned a plane
With joy your heart did burst

Boise and Vegas, Coalinga and Maine
You've traveled far and wide
Knowing you will be landing with
Your life long companion by your side

Yet as you grow older the focus becomes
How to beat the odds and stay alive
To prove yourself to be a true Pereira
And live to the age of 95

And so you share the news with us
Your decision to sell the plane
We feel so proud, you are so wise
Please know how we share in your pain

Yet each time we hear a news report
Where a small plane kissed the ground
We'll feel assured and quite content
Knowing you and Mom are still around

So what have you taught your children
By your legacy in the sky?
Be bold enough to chase your dreams
Yet wise enough to know when to say goodbye

Dad, you are my rock of Gibraltar!

I love you,

Sis

1/7/03—Cathy Update #33
(6 Days After LAST Chemo Treatment)

Happy New Year!

Ding dong the witch is dead, which old witch? The wicked witch!
(sing along: from the Wizard of Oz)

I feel like a munchkin with flowers growing out of my shoes. Finishing my last chemo treatment was like having the house land on my cancer, no more spinning and pitching. Like graduation day, no more homework and tests. Like finishing a marathon, no more cramps and feeling out of breath…well, maybe next week. The day after treatment I was walking on cloud nine, but by the next day I was more tired than ever. Obviously the cumulative effect of 8 treatments isn't going away just yet. Still, I relish the thought that this part is over! Radiation treatments last just 6 weeks, a spit in the bucket compared to 6 months. My New Year's resolution: To keep this attitude and appreciation of life I have developed from this experience. I don't want to lose sight of the insight I have gained. I do, however, want to lose sight of the weight I have gained. That's my second resolution.

My mom, Charlie and I walked into the chemo lounge last Thursday carrying chilled bubbly (alcohol free champagne and sparkling cider), Belgian chocolates and New Year party supplies. I walked around asking the patients and medical staff if they wanted a hat, a tiara or a lei (the Hawaiian version). You should have seen the face on some of the men. Of course they wanted to get laid (I tried spelling leied but spell check won't accept it). The atmosphere was jovial as the nurses, wearing their tiaras, served up chemo cocktails intravenously as we all sipped tall glasses of bubbly. In a strange way I'm going to miss it. I adore Ses, my favorite nurse, and told her so in the thank you card I gave her (the card shows a drawing of a butt with grass growing on it, opens to say "Mucho Grassy Ass."). I met so many incredible people on this journey. My faith in the human race has been rekindled. The people who work in this profession are saints.

138

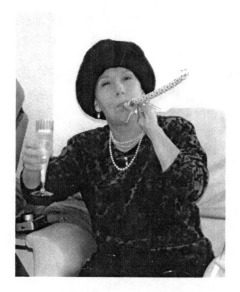

*New Year's celebration in the chemo lounge and my
last chemo treatment.*

Next step, radiation treatments (fried titty and nuked nipple) beginning the last week of January, Monday through Friday for 6 weeks. Treatments only last about 5 minutes, but driving to Stockton after work every day and then home again will make it seem longer. According to Vickie (one of the chemo lounge regulars now recovering from ovarian cancer after having breast cancer 2 years ago) radiation treatments aren't so bad. I'm just hoping to get my energy back soon. I'm so tired of being tired.

I visit my friend Michael at least once each week, not so much to lift his spirits, as to lift mine. He has such a Divine spirit. Joe (my friend, massage therapist, cancer survivor, etc.) is also friends with Michael. After hearing Michael complain about some of his home nurses' gloom and doom behavior, Joe recommended a sign be posted for his visitors. So I made that sign for Michael that says "Mike is not dying of cancer, he is living with it. Please act accordingly." Although Michael's doctor does not agree with us, Joe, Michael and I firmly believe that attitude and prayer can make liars out of doctors. That's our plan and we're sticking to it.

On New Years day my family celebrated our belated Christmas. This year we skipped the gift exchange between adults and only gave gifts to the children due to the economy's impact on our family. I decided that we really don't need to do a gift exchange even in the future, it seems so extravagant considering none of us 'needs' for anything. So, my family has agreed from now on we will be sponsoring a family for Christmas and provide presents to them instead of each other. Christmas will be so much more meaningful giving to a family who needs that extra help. What a wonderful lesson in charity for the children. Next year is going to be great!

This New Year holds so much promise. I walk forward to embrace what's ahead of me. My son's graduation, my wedding, moving to Paradise, house remodeling…so many things to look forward to. So much life yet to live!

And so the time has come for me to end my weekly update ramblings. You have heard from me once each week for six months now. What a ride it's been. I will send you occasional updates as I go through my radiation treatments and beyond, but will no longer keep the weekly pace. I could continue doing this for years, as I never seem to run out of things to talk about. I could become a weekly columnist yacking about the various topics that cross my life, yet I choose a different path.

Thank you for being there for me, an audience for whom to share my inner most thoughts. Thank you for inspiring me, for wanting to learn about the cancer experience so as to become more empathetic to others. Thank you for encouraging me to publish (Joan's group gave me "Publishing for Dummies" so appropriate for me) and I will let you know how that adventure turns out.

But most of all, thank you for caring enough to be there. Because of you, I am not only surviving, I am THRIVING!!

Bye for now,

cMc

1/19/03—Cathy Update #34 (Less Than 2 Weeks Later)

"Clowns to the left of me, jokers to the right, here I am…
stuck in the middle with you."
(Sing Along: Lyrics by Stealer's Wheel, Joe Egan & Jerry Rafferty)

If you remember that song, you are as old as I am. Ha! I feel like I am in limbo land, in the space between chemo and radiation treatments. Bits and pieces of normalcy are creeping back into my life, yet I must remind myself I'm not done yet and I still need to conserve my energy for it will take time for me to heal from all this.

I went on a business trip down to southern California this week. My partner Sheila and I drove down because you can't convince me it is safe to fly in an airplane with all those viruses swirling around in the re-circulated air. I was exhausted by the time I arrived home and will take the next week off to recuperate. Charlie's car is dying a slow and painful death (slow in time and painful on the pocket book). We decided to shop for a truck since we anticipate years of home improvements ahead of us. We have always been economy car owners, and we don't know what the truck we are doing. If you have any hints, please let us know.

I spent hours on the phone with our architect going over the elevations and blue prints on the remodel project last week. At one point, Charlie asked me a question about the blue prints while my mind was still stuck in truck mode. I lost it. I started to cry because my brain is not yet capable of doing the multi-subject juggling that was the norm in my previous life. I can't seem to shift gears from one project to the next without a "transition" period to switch over. I feel as if I've lost my mind, literally, and I can't wait for it to come back.

And So it Is Here in Limbo Land

I'm learning to cope with hot flashes. I haven't had a period in three months (who said chemo is a bad thing?) and I have the pleasure of experiencing menopause early as my ovaries became omelets months ago.

Fortunately my flashes are mild and you can recognize me in any restaurant. I'm the one who keeps taking her coat off, then put it on again, at 5 minute increments throughout the meal. I guess you can call it an "on again, off again affair." I've started following my weight watchers regime again. I noticed I have gained a pound each week this past month. Ouch. Now that I am finished with chemo it is easier for me to accept denial of comfort food and the pleasures of eating sweets. Psychologically I couldn't refuse before, somehow justifying my bad eating habits because I was "suffering" (truly psychologically based, as I can't honestly consider my cancer experience as suffering, thank God). Last night my friend Gayle and I went to see another friend Steve and his band at the School for the Deaf. They are the first, and only, Deaf band and they go by the name Beethoven's Nightmare. It was truly a Deaf cultural experience with fun visual effects and a guest mime from Russia (that's right, he's Deaf too) was incredible. I know you are thinking, "how can Deaf people enjoy music?" Some of the audience members held balloons so they could feel the vibrations of the drum and bass. There weren't many melodies, but plenty of clever background rhythms. Lyrics were done in sign language and there were lots of light tricks to provide a saturation of visual effects. During the last song they invited the audience to come up on stage and dance. Gayle and I were up there like a couple of groupies, dancing away on stage at a "rock concert." I must be feeling better.

I had my last weekly appointment with my oncologist last week and a strange thing happened…I felt sad. I am glad to be done with chemo treatments, but sad that I will miss the people I have developed a bond with after 6 months of weekly appointments. I have become particularly fond of Dr. Bangladesh, whose sense of humor kicked in after a few weeks of my humor abuse. He is not only kind and knowledgeable; he is respectful and kind to his staff. No ego problems here. You have to respect a doctor who drives a Honda Accord wagon (same car as mine) and who drives to Tracy once each week so his patients don't have to drive up to see him. As for Ses, my favorite RN and chemo cocktail waitress, she, Mom and I are going to lunch at Neiman Marcus in San Francisco next week to make up for the annual ritual I missed while "suffering" the stomach flu last December. I'm not letting go of her that easy.

I now understand why my chemotherapy treatments were given in 4 dose stages. The first dose was the most powerful, my body not knowing how to react, with the most severe side effects. The second dose less so. The third dose, even less yet. By the fourth dose, my body had adjusted and the side effects were much less. I imagine my body over time becomes strong enough to fight the effects of the chemo, which in turn makes it less effective in killing the bad boy cells (if I were to continue further treatments). With the exception of the fatigue factor, my last dose of Taxotere gave me no mouth problems what so ever. My hair continues to grow back and is beginning to get curly. I am, however, still losing hair in some spots, as I need to fill in the bald spots on my eyebrows now. Fortunately I still have a few lashes hanging in there, just enough to stick mascara to. When it's warm enough, I even feel bold enough to expose my salt and pepper butch hairdo to the world. It's amazing what huge earrings can do to complete the fashion statement.

One last bit of news that you may want to get in on. The security guards at my work have a "pinup" calendar for sale to raise funds for breast cancer research. I was reading the newspaper this week and saw a picture of Jason, one of my favorites, posing like a model (sorry girls, there is very little skin exposed in these pictures, but the faces and the cause are certainly worth the purchase). When I read the article and found out that the funds are being donated to breast cancer research my eyes teared up. Even though I know I am not the only person they know who has gone through this, every time I hear about events that support breast cancer I get very emotional. Just like the feeling of sisterhood that comes when meeting a total stranger who has also been through this. Cancer is very personal, yet so many people experience it, there is a sense of belonging to a special community. It's a strange phenomenon.

Next Wednesday is my appointment with the radiologist to get "targeted" for my radiation treatments. I'll be tattooed with little marks to make sure the machine lines up accurately for each of my daily treatments over the next 6 weeks. I'll fill you in with more info as I go through it.

Until you read again,

cMc

p.s. Michael (Cupcake) became a grandfather on January 14. Now, more than ever, he has inspiration to fuel his fight. He began a new chemotherapy treatment two weeks ago and seems to be getting his appetite back. Looks like he's on an upswing. Keep those prayers coming.

1/29/03—Cathy Update #35
(10 Days Later)

Michael Update

It is with mixed emotions that I share this information with you; sadness for the loss of an incredible human being, relief that his pain and suffering has ended.

Michael "Cupcake" Caraveo passed away this morning between 9-10:00 am from pneumonia and cancer related complications.

I will forward information about the memorial services as soon as I know.

He is at peace, for he found God during his cancer journey. He is in good hands.

He leaves a legacy through me, for the caring and giving way he lived his life will remain in my memory as long as I live and I will share the same with those around me so his light will never dim.

Thank you for all your prayers.

cMc

2/3/03—Cathy Update #36
(7th Day of Daily Radiation Treatments)

Let It Be

(sing along: lyrics by Paul McCartney and John Lennon)

And so the Universal plan plays it course and we don't understand why things happen. All we can do is…let it be.

I planned to write about my radiation treatments this week, but with the passing of Michael, and the Shuttle Columbia disaster (it broke apart upon landing), I find my focus more on recent events than on myself. There is still a light that shines on me, for this morning I awoke to be given a new day on this Earth. I found unprecedented energy flowing through me while I was helping Michael's daughter Kimmy this past week. I felt no fatigue for my focus was outside myself and channeled to support another in her time of need. I thank God for allowing me to be present. Perhaps this coming week, my second week of radiation treatments, I will become more tired, which is what is expected. But for now I am able to provide the attention that is needed in her hour of need.

Michael's passing brought to my attention how 'hope' could possibly get in the way. In hoping we will get better and avoiding planning for our demise, we neglect to provide the details needed to reduce the stress our loved ones experience while planning for the ceremony that follows our passing and tying up financial loose ends. I have a Will, but I don't have instructions written down for what I want to happen at my funeral. I don't have a list of who I want to give things to, heirlooms, jewelry, mementos, etc. that have sentimental value. My parents have a list of all their accounts, where everything is, who gets what, and as it changes they provide us updates (My anal retentive genes comes from both sides of my family). If only Michael had done the same, then Kimmy wouldn't be going through what she is faced with in these coming months. If only all of us would do the same so our children won't have to make these decisions at the mortuary, search through the house for files and records. If only our children and loved ones would have nothing to do but grieve.

I think people avoid this type of estate planning because they are afraid. Afraid to admit we are mortal and we may die at any time. But hey, cancer or no cancer, I could get hit by a Mack truck crossing the street any day. I could get hit by a stray bullet meant for a gang member or a sniper's bullet fired by a crazed lunatic seeking vengeance. I could get hit by falling space shuttle debris. But I don't live my life in fear that any of these things are going to happen.

It matters not how you die or when you die, but HOW you LIVE and WHEN you LIVE. Don't wait until you are diagnosed with an illness to discover the joy of appreciating every new day that dawns before you. Live life to the fullest, NOW!

Planning for your last days on Earth and the days afterward is not an admission that we are ready to leave. It is simply the single most precious gift we can give to our survivors to make their experience with our passing less stressful. Do it while you are healthy, get it over with, write it down, put it in the safe or safe deposit box, or give copies to everyone. Once it is done you can breathe a sigh of relief that it won't be a worry in the future, for you or for anyone. Hopefully that future is far, far away. And if, God forbid, you too are diagnosed with an illness that requires your undivided attention for spiritual energy to heal, at least you won't have to give up any of that 'hope' energy making plans for the "just in case" scenario we all dread while trying to heal our body and soul.

If you complete this task now, when the time comes and they ask themselves "what do I do now?" …there will be an answer …let it be.

cMc

p.s. Sorry for the lecture, these are simply words of wisdom. Now I need to go and practice what I preach.

2/13/03—Cathy Update #37
(15th Day of Radiation Treatments)

I suppose death is a part of most cancer survivor's journey. If it is not someone we meet while going through treatments, attending support groups and workshops, it may possibly be someone in the family by the natural turn of events in time. Most of us will experience a minimum of one to two years for treatment and recovery, some will take longer. Knowing someone who passes away during that period of time isn't unusual, yet how we react to it is now different. The most important lesson is to not let it derail us. Give all you have in your soul to support and console those in need, then move on and give all you have in your soul to persevere in your own journey of survival.

I'm in the Middle of My Third Week of Radiation Treatments.
Life Is Good!

My eyebrows are growing like crazy. I say "hello" to each new stray hair as I pluck it to keep my brow curve. If only my eye lashes would start growing back. I just barely have enough to put the mascara on. I no longer need to smother my face in cocoa butter every night. My body oils are coming back and my skin is less dry. I can wash my hair without looking at my hands to count the hairs that have fallen out. They aren't falling out any more, in fact, I have a full and thick head of curly, gray and black hair. I went from looking like my son's sister to looking like my mother's sister (because of the gray hair). Mom gets a big kick out of that. I don't wear my wig any more, just a hat to keep my head warm. Inside I wear nothing but my new hair, a symbol of my transition from ignorance to wisdom. This journey has changed me. I like me better now.

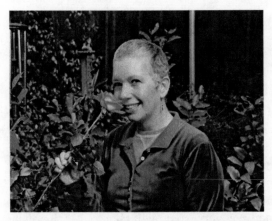

I finally have enough hair to go "natural" in public.

I'm stretching and exercising more each morning. My muscles are still slow to recover. My energy level the past 2 weeks has been fantastic. Charlie and I went to lovely Shelly's house for a Chinese New Year/open house/ birthday party last Saturday. We drank wine and stayed up past midnight, just like grown ups. On Monday I asked my radiologist, Dr. Goldfinger, when I was going to start feeling tired. I forgot to knock on wood. The very next day I started feeling the fatigue from my new treatments. Still nothing like chemo. My mind is clear, my creativity is coming back. I feel motivated again. I'm working 50% now and driving one hour to my radiation treatments every afternoon, Monday through Friday. For now, my energy level is quite acceptable.

I have 3 'X' markings on my chest (about 2 inches long) to line up the red laser beams that align the radiation machine known as a linear accelerator (cross my heart, hope to die, stick a needle in my eye. Who thinks up these things?). They were nice enough to give me the option for ink markings instead of permanent tattoos. I need to be re-marked every few days, but then, I'm used to people making remarks about me (re-marks…get it?). After each treatment, I apply Aquaphor healing ointment (yuck, it's like Vaseline) to my skin to keep it moist and prevent peeling. So far, after 13 treatments, I only have a slight coloration on my skin. No discomfort yet. My boob is slightly swollen (yippee) so I am very symmetrical, unfortunately that isn't permanent. Eventually I will shrink down again and become even smaller than before radiation treatment started (boo hoo, or would that be, boob who?). Fortunately, Cher and Cher-alike are small enough I don't need to wear a bra during treatment (gravity has little effect on itty bitty titties). Eventually it will become too painful to wear such a thing (such a sling) so I am wearing comfy tee shirts underneath another top to keep my skin from rubbing against my clothes.

I have new bosom buddies to chat with while waiting for treatments. I am terrible remembering names, so I refer to them by the time of their appointments and the machine they get zapped with. I am 3:30/old machine. According to 3:30/new machine, she didn't begin to experience discomforting burning until her 22nd treatment. That is 2/3 of the way through treatment. Today she told me of a blister under her arm and warned me to make sure I put the ointment high enough to cover the entire treatment area. My pal 3:45/old machine began experiencing fatigue last week, but I have been lucky to have lasted one week longer before feeling tired. Today the new machine broke down, so only us old machine patients received our treatments. So much for feeling bad that we are stuck with the Rambler model. Nothing wrong with something tried and true. Overall, compared to chemo treatments, this is a piece of cake so far.

My treatments only last about 5 minutes. I lay down on a slanted board adjusted specifically for me and place my hand behind my head and rest my elbow out. The technicians (excuse me, technologists) line up the red laser beams with the Xs on my chest. Once I am adjusted perfectly I can breath, but can't move out of place. They slip in a metallic board in front of the opening where the beam comes out (how is this for techie talk?). This "board" changes the shape of the beam so it curves with the shape of my breast. Then, they slip another hard plastic sheet in front of the "board" that holds a lead block shaped like my ribs. This prevents the beam from penetrating my rib and lung area. Initially, the "thing" (where the beam comes from) is above my head. The "thing" then rotates to my right side, about a 45 degree angle above my breast. The technologists then leave the room saying "here we go" (WE?) and the beam lasts for about 40 seconds. I don't feel a thing. Then the "thing" rotates to my left side and stops about 45 degrees under my breast. The lead shield is replaced with another one for this specific angle. I then receive another 40 second dose from this side. Once the dose is finished, I am free to move my arm back to a normal position. At first my arm would go numb, but now I'm getting used to it. The technologists move very quickly so that I don't have to suffer in that prone position too long.

That's all there is to it. One hour on the road for a 5 minute treatment, every day. It's a medical miracle. Never thought 5 minutes in a Rambler could be considered a blessing. When I feel the urge to make the drive more worth it, I stay and chat with 3:45/old machine or work the jigsaw puzzle in the waiting room. Mondays I see Dr. Goldfinger and every other Wednesday I have blood drawn. My counts are in the normal range. Go figure. Can't really categorize me as "normal."

Two friends have now introduced me to newly diagnosed cancer patients. I find myself in the counseling mode, on the other side of the coin, helping others begin their journeys. I will try my best to bring to them the spirit of hope and the understanding of how to experience this as a "bump in the road" and keep their spirits up to persevere. As Olivia and I discussed earlier this week, the cancer journey has two inter-twining paths, one is medical and the other is spiritual. We don't experience one without the other. They go hand in hand. Medicine alone may not be enough to cure and sometimes the human spirit (holy spirit?) can cure all on it's own. Such is the miracle of life.

May you be with the one you love on Valentine's Day.

"And if you can't be with the one you love, honey, love the one you're with."

(sing along: lyrics by Steven Stills)

Happy Valentine's Day!

cMc

p.s. "love the one you're with" platonically of course, silly. This isn't the 60's.

3/3/03—Cathy Update #38
(26th Day of Radiation Treatments)

Two Weeks More Then I'm out the Door!

The light at the end of the tunnel is so bright, I have to wear shades. These past 5 weeks of radiation treatments have been a breeze. I have only slight discomfort, like a sunburn, on the left half of my chest as the treatments cover my entire left breast and lymph gland area under my arm. Starting Tuesday they will change the focus of the beams to just the areas where my tumor and lymph nodes were removed for my last 8 treatments. I will transfer over to the new machine (the Ferrari) for these more precise treatments (By the way, the "thing" where the beam comes from that I referred to in my last update is called a 'columnator' which rotates on the end of the 'gantry'). I don't know what to expect during these last few weeks, but I can endure anything knowing how close I am to completion.

March 12, the day before my last treatment, Papa Smurf will remove Cathy-ter (the port inserted for my chemo treatments). It's an office procedure so I won't need to go into the hospital. I don't even notice her any more she is so comfortable and out of the way. In a strange way, I'm going to miss her (having 3 boobs is novel). Located on my lower right rib, I guess this is what Adam felt like. His rib gave life to Eve. The port on my rib gave life to me.

Irony! After my blood counts returned to mid-normal range, I caught a cold. I don't now whether it's because I let down my guard and started touching doorknobs again or because I am working 50%-time now and interact with more people. Either way, I count my blessings I didn't catch it while my blood counts and energy were low. Even with this cold I feel fantastic!

I was watching an episode of Scientific American (Alan Alda hosts this fascinating series on PBS) that focused on the Placebo Effect. It's amazing how people can 'believe' themselves into healing without medicine. A friend also talked with me about her sister, diagnosed with cancer and given little chance of survival, who is now 9 years cancer free. Her story is a true reminder of how the human spirit can overcome illness, despite the odds. As grateful as I am for the medical marvels that have healed me, I am even more grateful for the spiritual miracle granted to me during my journey. I try to keep this in mind to guide me, for I have a new challenge, not within myself, but for my son.

Paul developed a lump in a lymph node under his jaw last December. At first, we believed it to be Cat Scratch, as a cat scratched him weeks before and he is allergic. The doctor thought it to be a blocked salivary gland (just like a kidney stone or gall stone). He took antibiotics for 10 days, to no avail. A CT scan proved it to be a lymph node, and a needle core biopsy was done. Results were inconclusive. Three more weeks of stronger antibiotics haven't helped much. It is pretty much the same size, about an inch in diameter. Next step…surgery. I am fine when I don't think about it, but I can work myself into such a whirlwind of worry if I dwell on it too long. I have had nothing but positive energy surrounding my cancer experience yet as a mother, I can't help but fall into worry about my son, my baby. Funny how it hurts worse when it is your child than when it is yourself. *(It turned out that Paul did indeed have Cat Scratch and the lump slowly dissolved over several months, without surgery)*

Please keep Paul in your prayers and surround him with the same positive energy you sent my way. Pray for Cat Scratch or some other benign ailment that will lead to hatred of clawed animals (sorry cat lovers) and not a new journey down my path. Pray for Murphy's law, the hassle of surgery just to find out it was "nothing." Pray that I am strong enough to keep the same positive energy surrounding Paul during his medical procedures that I was able to sustain during my own.

Meanwhile, life continues down the path of my future. The recent rains brought some of the most beautiful rainbows I have ever seen. Serendipitous as they hang above the Cancer Center on my drive to treatments in the afternoon. Spring-cleaning is afoot, purging the old, preparing for garage sales that are inevitable when we blend our two households into one this coming summer. We are gardening a plenty in our little Garden of Eden in Paradise. Dieting is once again on hold, Valentine 's Day and now Girl Scout cookies are ensuring I won't begin my Weight Watchers regime until later. Perhaps it's better that I wait until I am completely done with treatments before I begin to "deny" myself the pleasures of frivolous food.

We refinanced the house with cash out to begin our remodeling (certain to become a 10-year project). I ordered new eye glasses, with hip, cool frames to match my new shorter hairdo. I finished sewing projects started pre-surgery and neglected during the motivation-less chemo phase. I finished my new belly dance belt, complete with Pakistani coins, to wear now that my hips are gearing up to dance again. I am planning to participate in future cancer events. More info later about the Surviving Beautifully fashion show in April and the Relay for Life cancer fundraiser in May.

I find myself conflicted between my worry for Paul and my exhilaration about my new life and my newfound level of energy. I guess this is proof that all journeys are filled with ups and downs. Life isn't life without the range of feelings that make us human. Good and bad, happy and sad...life goes on.

Caio for now.

cMc

3/4/03—Cathy Update #39
(The Next Day)

Paul Update

Talk about Murphy's Law! No sooner do I send out my update of 3/3/03, mentioning my worry about Paul's lump, then good news comes our way. Wow, I am amazed at how fast prayer works. I'm also a little embarrassed I spoke too soon. (I learned how to worry from my mom. I call it "premature worry syndrome.")

We had an appointment yesterday with the surgeon to schedule Paul's operation. Upon examination, the surgeon feels the lump and notices it has become smaller. He takes another needle biopsy and suggests we wait a few more months to see if the lump subsides even more before considering surgery.

Thank you, thank you, thank you. Once again, you came through for me.

Have an absolutely wonderful day!!!

cMc

3/13/03—Cathy Update #40
(A Few Days After Last Radiation Treatment)

Haaaaaaaaallelujah!
Haaaaaaaaallelujah!
Hallelujah,
Hallelujah,
Halleeeeeeeeelujah!

I can hear the phat lady sing! (fat is soooo last century)

9 months of treatment, I should be giving birth. I am! Birth to a new life!

My treatments are over, done with, finished, completed, terminated.

Finish, pah!
Finito
Kaput

Time for a Martini. No, Make That Tee Martoonees

Here I sit, bright red burned boob on the left, stitches on my ribs to the right (Cathy-ter was removed yesterday. I'm going to make a necklace out of it). So, what ever you do, don't hug me! Love me from afar. Despite my condition, I FEEL MAWVELOUS! Celebrate with me tonight, with a prayer for all of those walking this same path, that they will soon reach this day where it is all behind us.

"I'm comin' up so you better get this party started"…Pink!
(sing along: performed by Pink)

Did someone say party? Yes, that would be my good buddy Sue Eadie. She will be the hostess of the best darn post-cancer treatment party of the year. I'll give you details later about dates and times of at least two celebrations (one East Bay and one Valley) that will happen in the next few months. Meanwhile…

…please consider joining me at the Surviving Beautifully (Celebrating Life's Magic) Fashion Show on Sunday April 13 at 2:00pm at the Stockton Radisson. This is a fun event sponsored by St. Joseph's Regional Cancer Center where cancer survivors model not only beautiful fashions, but also new attitudes towards living. I'll be one of the models and will be modeling my latest dance costume creation (painstakingly sewn during my cancer journey) as well as my newest jewelry acquisition, the Cathy-ter necklace. There will be a champagne reception immediately following the show. Also, a silent auction and door prizes will add to the value of your $10 ticket. Tickets are available through me, so please let me know if you want to join us.

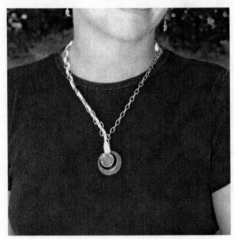

This is the necklace I made out of the port and catheter that I received my chemo treatments through.

And so, I celebrate the end of the "formal" treatment phase. I will still follow up with a 5 year regiment of Tamoxifen, but this will be no different than taking birth control pills every day (I've heard someone call them the "bitch" pills. Charlie is hoping my reaction will be different than that. The first 5 years of marriage should be better than that). This medication will prevent estrogen from reaching cancer cells while it allows estrogen to reach my bones so I will be less likely to develop osteoporosis. Since my tumor was estrogen-receptor positive, we don't want any estrogen to re-grow another tumor.

Here I am. I've had a lot of time these past 9 months to think. What is the point of all this? Here is my theory.

The Point!

I believe a little of both camps, the one that says life is all fate and the one that says we have complete control over it. I believe fate deals us the major events in our lives, yet it is our choice how to react to these events that helps to shape our future. If we continually choose to contribute positively to the natural flow of energy that is our universe, we will eventually have a positive affect on our future. If we continually choose to leave a path of destruction and negative energy by our reaction to these events, then "shit happens." It's simple. It's the difference between good and evil, God and Devil (ever notice there is only one letter difference!). It's not that hard to figure out.

I believe (and so does science) that every one, every body gets cancer. Some are able to destroy it with their own immune systems and thus it never becomes an obstruction to life. Some of us aren't so lucky. So what can we do to stack the odds in our favor? How can we behave so our immune systems will be better able to destroy cancer? Drink Barley grass juice? Eat your vegetables? Become vegetarians? Don't breath air pollution? Exercise? Pray? Meditate? Slow down? Why not all of them? Why not try just one? Cancer me once, shame on you. Cancer me twice, shame on me.

What's the point? The point is I've been given a second chance. A wake up call. The poor souls who die instantly from accidents don't get a second chance. Those who get cancer at least have time (for some it may not be long, but it's amazing how much life you can live in a brief time). If I have only a few more years left, I will live them so preciously and so aware because of this journey. This is the point. If I have 60 more years, the same applies.

What's the point? Don't wait until you get cancer to get the point! Do a little preventative maintenance. MAKE your second chance.

Work at a job you love. Work with people you like. Love your family, and if you don't, find a way to. Love your body. When they say "your body is a Temple" they mean treat it with the same respect you give the Temple, Church, what ever. Love yourself. Love your fellow man (or sister woman). Love God. Love Life!

John and Paul were right! "All you need is love."

cMc

4/10/03—Cathy Update #41
(1 Month After Last Radiation Treatment)

Pack and Purge

My Life Is in Boxes.

Many cancer survivors have new perspectives that lead to new lives and lifestyles. Even before my cancer, I was planning a new life with Charlie. Our department at work was reorganized and the last year has been constant with change and movement, most of which I was absent for. Last Friday I found myself sitting in my office, reading an e-mail that said "the office moves planned for April 10th have been cancelled." Cancelled in RED letters. Any other day… any other time… any other life…my response would have been, "whatever." Instead, for me, this message brought uncontrollable tears.

Have I been TOO upbeat about my cancer journey? Did I forget to cry enough? Is that where the tears came from? Perhaps it's because I'm tired, doing too much, not ready for this pace of life I left 10 months ago. I've been working in the same office for 10 years (unheard of in our circles and the culture of my work place) and I've been anticipating moving to a new office since before my surgery. I've been waiting, looking forward to a change that hasn't come yet. I've also been waiting for years to begin my new life with Charlie. Waiting until Paul graduates from high school. 5 years of dreaming, planning, anticipating. I felt like the rug was pulled out from under me when I read that e-mail. How dare they prevent me from moving on! After much analysis (cheaper than a therapist) I think I figured it out.

Cancer Survivors Need to Grieve!!

We need to grieve what we have left behind. For some, it's a part of the body. For many, it's a lifestyle and way of looking at the world. For all of us, it's our change in attitude toward life. For me, EVERYTHING IS CHANGING!

I have lived in my current house for 10 years. I am surrounded by boxes as I plan for the upcoming neighborhood block sale and eventual move during the summer. I'm leaving my support system that has provided my son and me with a safety net for this single mother with a career. Mary (my next door neighbor) was always there to pick up Paul when I couldn't get to school in time. She was the keeper of the extra key for the many times we locked ourselves out. I have worked in my office for 10 years with a group of 'friends' that has been disbanded by the reorganization. A new boss, a new boss's boss, and a new boss's, boss's boss. I really don't know what to expect as I have grown comfortable with my style of working. I am in boxes there too. Paul is a senior in high school. He starts college next year. My boy is now a man.

I need to take the time to cry for what I am leaving behind...a neighborhood, colleagues, a child, and the old Cathy. I have been so enthralled by the excitement of my new life and the positive changes that lay ahead; I have forgotten to grieve what I am leaving.

It was hard. I'm still teary eyed as I write this. I found instant gratification with the clearance rack at Gottchalks as I chose to suppress my tears. That worked for a few days. I couldn't eat chocolate or drink excessively as I'm currently faithful to the Weight Watchers program, at least for now. I'm back in my tai chi class and other than the occasional tear, I am handling the stress much better than I used to. As my dearest Olivia would say, "too blessed to be stressed."

Speaking of blessings...Paul's lump has faded away! Thank you for your prayers and for constantly asking me how he is doing. One less McClain to worry about, two less when you think about it.

I'm preparing for the Surviving Beautifully fashion show on Sunday. Not only will I be wearing the costume I designed and created, I'll be dancing and signing (that's signing, not singing) as I wiggle my ass all over the runway. I don't usually pay that much attention to "beauty" and making myself "all perty" but one thing I noticed as I am doing my manicure is my fingernails have a distinct line between the "chemo" nail and the "post-chemo" nail. About half of my fingernails are slightly brownish and the newer half is pink and healthy. That's a Taxotere trait I never noticed before, but then again, I rarely pay any attention to that kinda stuff. My hair is also in a transition stage. Half my hair is old and the other half is still growing back, so I'm keeping it short for now until it's all behaving the same.

It's a time of transition. Not just for me, but for many.

Until I write again, let's all say a prayer for world peace and the safety of all people involved in political strife, no matter where.

cMc

4/18/03—Cathy Update #42
(5 Weeks After Last Radiation Treatment)

Surviving Beautifully!! (And the Signing Survivor Seder)

The Surviving Beautifully fashion show was incredible. I bonded with 41 cancer survivor models ranging from ages 10 to 84. One of the best benefits of meeting these people is realizing how many of them have survived cancer not just once, but twice! This brings relief should the unthinkable happen and my cancer returns. I have never felt so welcomed, so supported, so much like "I belong" before spending the day with these wonderful people.

Over 500 guests participated in the silent auction and raffle prizes, watched their loved ones modeling clothes from home or from local stores displaying Spring fashion, and joined in the champagne reception (except I opted for the beer, GREAT microbrew from Kelley's brewery in Manteca). The purpose wasn't to model the clothes, but to model the attitude of survival in the face of cancer. For me, it was like a graduation ceremony celebrating the end of my treatments. Mom, Charlie, Paul, Sherry and my buddy John were there. The "signing Seybold sisters" came and my friend (and right hand at work) Sheila brought her sister-in-law. Yet the most important guest who came was my mom's friend Alice, over 40 years a cancer survivor and one hell of a great lady.

The biggest lesson I learned that day…LIFE IS AN IMPROVISATION! No matter how well you plan your life, no matter how perfect the rehearsal, when "real life" happens, God throws you a curve ball and watches to see how you handle it (perhaps that is why "reality TV" is so popular. People relate to the unpredictable). It's not the curve of the ball that counts, its how we handle it. So it is with cancer…and on Sunday, so it was for my "performance."

In front of an audience of over 500 (although the most forgiving and supportive audience there could ever be) my perfect, flawless, well rehearsed and choreographed dance and sign routine turned into a comedy routine. Somehow the audio tape (42 seconds in the middle of No Doubt's "Hey Baby" song) was taped over and after two attempts to wow the audience by unveiling my belly dance costume and beginning my dance, I ran to the sound engineer, fiddled with the tape, vowed to the audience that I would return soon, and ran out of the room.

The element of surprise was gone. The opportunity to wow them with a perfect routine was gone. The opportunity to do improv comedy had arrived. Yet, instead of feeling complete dread, I was somehow comforted by the fact that every single person surrounding me understood what it is like to need support while carrying a curve ball, and they refused to allow me to carry it alone. After realizing that my rehearsal tape was still at home (mistake number one) and I didn't have a back up tape (mistake number two) one of the other models spoke up, "I have that No Doubt CD in my car. Want me to get it?" Mysterious ways indeed!!

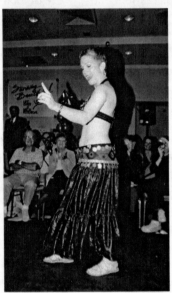

Fourth time's a charm. Dancing and signing at the Surviving Beautifully Fashion Show.

As the song played, I danced around with my veil for a full minute, making it up as I went along as I had no choreography for this part of the song. When I arrived at the part of the song I had rehearsed, I did not perform as flawlessly as originally planned, but that didn't matter any more (besides, no one else knew what the heck I was doing anyway). What mattered? Everyone in the audience was elated I had "survived" this little curve ball. Anticipation levels were high after so many false starts; no one will forget my name after I had been introduced 3 times. Not only did I still have the chance to entertain, but I had so much more time than originally planned. As in my cancer experience, I felt the hands that helped me carry the curve ball. "Its how you handle it," and I didn't have to handle it alone.

To continue in the spirit of surviving, I hosted my first Seder on Wednesday (On the first night of Passover, the Seder ceremony and meal commemorate the Jews freedom from slavery in Egypt). This was a particularly meaningful evening for me. I call it the Signing Survivor Seder because either sign language and/or cancer survivorship were common links between my guests. Only three of us were Jewish (and I'm only Jewish by injection) and my other guests were Christian, so the ceremony was particularly educational. I also refer to it as my "last supper" as it will be my last dinner party in my Tracy home before moving (I say that as if I had many, but this was only the second dinner party I had in 10 years. The hostess with the mostest I'm not). Ironically, Jesus' last supper was also a Seder and everyone there eventually became Christians. Go figure! By the end of the evening, we too had a total of 13 people in attendance. One difference though, we sat around the table, as opposed to all sitting on one side like in the painting.

The following morning began with our neighbor Mary and her 4 kids chasing their bunny rabbit in our front yard. Charlie and I joined in, then Joe next door. How fitting that we be chasing a bunny during Easter season. It was so much fun!! Don't forget to enjoy life's simplest pleasures. I'm going to miss this place. I'm going to miss the people…and the bunny.

I began taking my Tamoxifen every day and so far, I don't like it. I am hoping the symptoms will subside, or that perhaps what I am experiencing is from something else. I feel a bit anxious, like I used to the day or two before my menstrual cycle (still don't have those…yipee!). Perhaps it's just my hormones getting adjusted. I know these pills are going to help prevent a reoccurrence of my cancer. I simply long to feel "normal" the way I did before. Perhaps that is not possible, at least not for the next 5 years. Perhaps I am just obsessing about it (oh no! A bit of the old me coming back).

Have a wonderful Passover and/or a happy hoppy Easter (or as Ruthy says… East-over).

cMc

5/5/03—Cathy Update #43
(2 Months After Last Radiation Treatment)

Feliz Cinco de Mayo!!

I have this song from an old commercial stuck in my head. "What a difference a day makes… 24 little hours." The song probably came from some movie in the 1950s, like so many songs in commercials when I was growing up. Now I must be old because they play Led Zepplin songs in commercials now. I'm just grateful my son knows who Paul McCartney is and I actually found him playing my Jethro Tull vinyl on the record player a few months ago (If you recognize these groups, you're old too!).

What the heck (you are mumbling under your breath) does this have to do with anything? Well, if 24 hours can make such a difference that someone wrote a song about it, then I want to write a symphony about the past two weeks (again you mumble…oh no, another long e-mail update. Symphony?!).

It has been several weeks since I first began taking Tamoxifen pills daily and I feel quite normal again. At first I felt anxious, on the verge of crying all the time, feeling aches and pains all over. Thank heavens for time and the body's amazing ability to adapt. With the exception of a constant discomfort in my arm's lymph system (my own fault for not stretching and strengthening enough), I am now building up my strength as I begin to exercise more. When I do my stretches, my muscles give and don't fight back. My nose is getting reacquainted with my knee. For the first time since my first chemo treatment 10 months ago, I FEEL NORMAL! (well, within my definition any way). No chemo after taste. No bouts of fatigue. These past few days I have been stretching it a bit further, do a little more, and I am bouncing back. What a difference 2 weeks makes. Of course, my Charlie is after me constantly to take breaks and rest, so I am not permitted to over do it (I did have what I thought was a minor set back, but was nothing. The site where Cathy-ter was removed became inflamed. It was just a suture abscess, and once my body spit out the bitty piece of thread, I was all better). I just feel so good, I can't stop myself. I'm gardening and dancing like a maniac (or as studio Bob would say, a "lymph-o-maniac.")

It's that time of year again, when I pull out the last 12 months of day planners and gather my input for my performance appraisal (For those of you who are self employed, times like these are the reason you are self employed. You got it good!). I realized that I was diagnosed with cancer just 10 days into this 12 month review period, and yet I was amazed at how much I was able to accomplish. Thanks to the support of a great staff (Carol and Sheila, I can't do without you) my Disabilities Services Program survived, no… it thrived. This is one of God's little lessons in life, I AM expendable. And so, I choose not to work as much as I used to, because it appears I am more productive at work when I'm gone. I asked my boss if I can reduce my work schedule down to 70 percent-time beginning in August. I keep my fingers crossed that it will be approved. Life is too short to spend it working too hard for someone else.

When I was a teenager, my concept of "life span" was infinity. I was immortal and no matter what I did, how dangerous I lived, I would survive. Then, as I became a parent, I began to see life in cycles, parenthood, grandparenthood, etc. When I was taking care of my great-aunt Clara, elder care issues brought me down to earth and I began to think of my life span as being 85-95 years. Then cancer arrived. Now I see the possibility that my life span may be 45 to 50 years (and then again, it may be 95). Key words here "may be" and "possibility." I don't hold the key to the box where the answer lies, but I do get to decorate the box while it's closed. For me success will be defined by my ability to balance the need to plan for a comfortable future with the absolute requirement that I enjoy the present.

While sitting in the garage, watching the rain quench the garden out front, it came to me. Charlie and I are not remodeling a house, we are creating a sanctuary. As the first construction project begins, I also choose to spend more time in my garden (thank you Olivia for this metaphor) and it is there that I find such peace and tranquility. This, I am sure, will have a positive impact on my life span.

And speaking of construction…it's a good thing my strength is back so I could survive going through the process to get those plans approved. I spent several hours in the county permit office, going from window 5 to window 11 then to room 101 then back to window 5 then the cashier then back to window 5 again. After standing in lines between Mr. Pencil In-my-ear and an adult version of Charles Schultz's Pig Pen (boots all muddy, standing in a pile of dust on the carpet) I finally heard the words I was waiting for, "We'll call you when they are ready." Well, actually, I was hoping for different words. That didn't matter, what mattered to me that day was I was witnessing the beginning of my future (great song lyrics by Semisonic, "Closing time—every new beginning comes from some other beginning's end.").

I feel so excited these days, I can't figure out if it is pure joy of recovery, or a reaction to the Tamoxifen. You know how they give amphetamines to kids who are hyperactive and they respond by calming down? Well, they warned me about Tamoxifen and how I may become depressed, yet the opposite is happening. Maybe I am A.D.D. after all. That explains a lot!

Perhaps I am feeding off the energy I get while working toward my dreams. The Surviving Beautifully Fashion show broke a barrier for me by allowing me to overcome my obsession for perfection. I find myself flooded with creative ideas about sign language and dance, of writing and spreading my message of cancer survival. Initially, I didn't want to become a cancer campaigner, yet I find myself going in that direction. I am working on a tribute to fundraisers that I will be doing at the Tracy Relay for Life on Saturday May 17. I have prepared a 2 minute narration over music that will play while I dance on stage. The words express my appreciation for all the walkers' efforts in raising funds for research that made my treatment process successful. They will be able to see with their own eyes the energy that radiates from me, after only 2 months since my last treatment. I can't wait to thank everyone for all they have done for me, and others. I am also going to do a presentation at work during our Cancer Awareness Campaign. After talking with someone about the topic of cancer prevention, within "24 little hours" I had a rough draft of an outline for my talk "Who's on first?" which details some of my experiences and the importance of putting ourselves first when it comes to health matters.

I didn't plan to take this path, but here I am, and it feels right.

Despite the cancer stories unfolding around me (Pat's daughter's reoccurrence, Catherine's reoccurrence, Jim's wife's diagnosis, all 3 within the last two weeks) I still feel the need to stand on the highest mountain and rejoice. I know it is in the valley that I grew, but it's so nice to be back up on the mountain again.

Relay for life, May 17-18, 10:00 am to 10:00 am, Tracy High School stadium.

Update to follow.

cMc

5/18/03—Cathy Update #44
(10 Weeks After Last Radiation Treatment)

Relay for Life

What an incredible experience. Surrounded by a community working hard to rid our society of cancer, I too feel compelled to campaign to increase fundraising for cancer research. The Relay for Life event at the Tracy high school stadium this weekend is one of the largest events of its kind in Northern California. The concept began in 1985 in Tacoma Washington and today almost 3300 Relays occur annually raising over 245 million dollars for the American Cancer Society. Last year Tracy raised $272,000. This year we hope to top $300,000.

Beginning at 10:00 am on Saturday and ending at 10:00 am on Sunday these "24 little hours" are packed with empowering words, memorial events, food, fun, entertainment, education and fundraising events including raffles and silent auction. As 119 teams of 12-24 members kept at least one member from each team walking around the track for the entire event, the tents and vendors on the in field buzzed with activity. The entertainment was diverse with hip hop dance, scavenger hunt, rock music, people bingo, and numerous other musical genres represented. There were also special dress up laps including themes of crazy hats, patriotic, sports fanatic, tropical, twins, superhero and more. We began with a survivor's lap where all of us survivors wore purple Relay for Life shirts as we walked around the track to the applause of all those surrounding us. It felt incredible to get so much adulation for beating cancer. I walked arm-in-arm with my signing sister Linda as the sun shined, the wind blew and our souls soared.

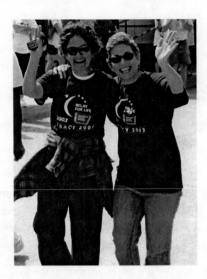

My bosom buddy Linda and I during the survivor's lap at Relay for Life.

After returning to our starting point, I quickly slipped into the tent to change into my dance costume while the "care givers" lap commenced. These past two weeks I have been tirelessly piecing together a special tribute including voice narration dubbed over music and choreography. I finally had the opportunity to thank everyone, in my own unique way, for all their efforts to raise money for cancer research. As the care givers lap ended and the teams began their relay, I entered the stage for my tribute of thanks. I've had this idea in my head since a week or two after my surgery. I envisioned dancing to music while my voice unveiled the story of my diagnosis and treatment. I talk about my fears of developing lymphedema and my subsequent elation due to recent breakthroughs and improvements in treatment. In the end, the music stops and while signing I say, "Thanks to your fundraising efforts for cancer research, you saved my job, you saved my joy, you saved my life. Thank you!"

This is just the beginning. I was asked to do a repeat tribute performance for the Lodi Relay for Life in June. Perhaps I can do others. I have a feeling this may also be a very effective fundraising tool. I hope to develop this into a 60 second Public Service Announcement and reach more people (in the words of Jabez, "enlarge my territory"). We often see fundraising requests, but how often to we hear 'thank you' from survivors? As survivors we constantly thank our family and friends, care givers and health professionals. I want to thank people who have donated money to improve the life of total strangers.

These past two weeks have been filled with lessons. I didn't realize what an ostrich (head in the sand) I was before my cancer journey. It seems I am more in tune with the unfolding of events around me. I 'listen' to words of wisdom, and 'recognize' them as such. I used to think I was in complete control of my destiny. I now realize that I am not in control of the direction of the path ahead of me, only the manner in which I travel that path. When I asked my dance instructor Nanna for her advice on improving the choreography of my tribute she said, "It doesn't matter what you do, but 'how' you do it is everything!" She didn't change one piece of my choreography, but she gave me tips on technique. "Keep your body grounded (knees bent, hips tucked forward, be balanced). Stretch your chest out, head towards heaven, shoulders down showing calmness. Slow down! Follow through with your movements, don't cut them short preparing for the next move." I not only choose to apply these tips to my movement in dance, but also as I move in my journey through life. Two years ago, I wouldn't have been aware enough to recognize this advice for the gift of wisdom it is. Life is but a dance. Spend more time dancing and less time worrying about the steps… we aren't the choreographer.

Friday night Barnes and Nobles (in Tracy, never-the-less) had a workshop on how to get published. Three local authors talked about marketing techniques, how to get a literary agent, and trying to land a deal with one of the "big houses" in New York with the "00" zip code. After hearing about the amount of work involved with getting a manuscript published, I was a bit turned off by the idea of publishing my updates. I want to share my experiences (as those of you who have been long term readers are quite aware) yet I am not sure that I want to devote tremendous amounts of energy trying to get published. Perhaps I can make a modest attempt, and if someone takes interest, then it is meant to be. If not, then that must not be the path chosen for me. What do you think about "Cathy Updates: A Year in the Life of my Breast Cancer Journey" for the title of the book? Anyone happen to know any literary agents in New York?

I don't know when I am going to write to you again. The anniversary of my diagnosis is June 12. Perhaps that would be the opportune time to finally sign off (no pun intended). By then you will have endured one year of updates from me. Maybe I should prepare a special tribute to all of you for your encouragement and inspiration that fueled my writing creativity. Alas with e-mail we have only words. Sign language, music and dancing (my favorite forms of expression) don't translate without high speed lines, Quick-time video and mega memory computers. My anniversary date is several weeks away yet, and if anything, you know how many words I can generate in that period of time. I'll do my best to write up something that can come close to expressing the gratitude I have for your attention this past year.

Until I write again,

Thank YOU!

cMc

6/12/03—Cathy Update #45 (1 Year Since Diagnosis)

My Final Update

One year ago today I heard that word "malignant" over the phone from my doctor while I was at work. I ran to my office, my side-kick Carol in tow. There she held me as I cried. That was the first of my many experiences of support through my cancer journey. I did not travel this path alone. I am thriving, one year later, because of all of you.

I sit here in my home office/sewing room/exercise room typing at the computer that has become my tool for written expression. Hard to believe that 14 years ago my good friend Fug (at the time my secretary) was explaining to me how unprofessional it sounded for me to include the phrase "we talked and talked and talked" in my monthly status report. Today, she pulled me aside as I walked down the hall and asked for my help in finding a good term to describe her "sub-sub category." Eventually the word "component" came out of me, not that it originated from inside of me, perhaps yet another bit of divine inspiration that has possessed me through this journey. Her request for my help meant so much to me (considering she used to correct my poor writing skills). Next week I submit my first essay to a writing contest. "Excerpts from Cathy Updates" includes two of my updates 7/23/03 and 7/27/03, edited slightly so they can stand alone. Thanks to all of you, I actually believe I am a good writer. I can't even begin to tell you how good it feels to hear your encouragement. You inspire me!

My son is downstairs right now with a motley crew of manly men, playing video games and acting rowdy. Tomorrow is his last day of high school. My baby graduates from high school on Saturday. So many of his friends are going into the Armed Forces. Others are going to a different college and staying in Tracy while we move away and start a new life with Charlie. He leaves behind all his friends, everything he has known for the past 10 years (except for me, although at this age, I think he enjoys his independence from me more than anything). I am not the only one arriving at a crossroad in life.

My request to work part-time was approved. Beginning in August I will be working 3 days a week. It's a huge relief to know I can retain at least one part of my life that I have known. This is more than just a job to me, it is an institution in which I have been integrally woven for 23 years. I'm not ready to leave, especially now when we have leadership I believe in. Working part time will make my commute (2 hours one way) more tolerable as I plan to drive to work on Tuesday, stay Tuesday and Wednesday nights with my parents and drive home after work on Thursday. It also gives Charlie and I a chance to adapt to living together. For 5 years we have been gone from each other 5 days a week and together for two. Now we reverse the order as we assimilate our lives. Now I will have more time to pursue a more relaxed lifestyle, nurture my creativity and yes, most probably, write some more.

Although I choose to no longer write about my cancer journey, I will forever include my lessons learned and divinely inspired insights in everything I write. Maybe I'll write about "My Remodeled Life" with a focus on the many remodeling projects ahead of us and including the joys and lessons found when starting a new life and a new marriage, the second time around. Let me know if you would be willing to be my victim again for this new line of subject matter. Having an audience to write to sure helps motivate me to sit down and write.

Although I choose to no longer write about my cancer journey, I embrace the idea of sharing my story with others. My first presentation about my cancer experience is 12 days away. I'll be talking to an audience of coworkers for our Cancer Awareness Campaign. Who knows where that may lead me? Well, I know who knows, but I'm not privy to that information at this time.

So I close this chapter of my life with my body healed, my heart filled with love, my mind bursting with creative energy and my soul at peace. Who would have ever thought that something as terrible as cancer could bring such a blessing to one's life? Well, I know who knew, and today, I know too!

With all my love,

cMc

My Charmed Life

Early in my cancer journey I was given the most precious gift of a charm shaped in a cross and blessed by the Pope. I am not a religious person and I no longer consider myself Catholic. Joan, a woman I only know as a business acquaintance, was thinking of me while visiting Italy and specifically chose the cross to have it blessed for me (someone she hardly knew). I was so touched by that loving deed. I was so taken by her kindness.

This charm sparked the beginning of my collection of charms for a bracelet commemorating my cancer journey. Through out the year documented in my updates, I looked for charms that symbolized the events and experiences surrounding me. Here is my list describing the meaning behind each of the charms on my bracelet.

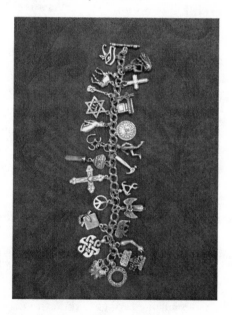

: The charms on my bracelet are listed below in order from top to bottom, first the left column then the right column.

173

Top Left

Udjat Eye: The Sacred Eye, an Egyptian symbol that represents God. My dear friend Nantz lives in France, and I miss her so much. She and I both got our tattoos at the same time (years ago), mine of a rose with a Celtic knot stem, and hers is the eye of Udjat. This charm reminds me of my love for her and her visit to me while I was going through radiation treatments. It also represents my new found connection to a more spiritual life.

Camel: I purchased this camel while attending the annual Rakkasah Middle Eastern dance festival in March. The camel is a symbol not only of this event, but a reminder of my love for belly dance. The license plate on my car (a camel colored station wagon) says "my camel" because I schlep so much stuff from here to there in my nomadic life.

Guitar: I picked this charm up in San Francisco the weekend of the Blues Festival. It represents my new-found patience for attending these blues events with Charlie. I also think of him when ever I see it, since he is "one with the Blues."

Star of David with chai symbol: When I first put the Pope cross on my charm bracelet, that was the only thing on the chain. This symbol signifies Christianity, yet I am not Christian. I added the Star of David to represent Judaism, Charlie's faith and that of many of my friends. As people of many religions were praying for me, I wanted to represent religious diversity on my bracelet as well.

Cat: This charm reminds me of my son's battle with "Cat Scratch." I'll never forget the decision we had to make while I was going through radiation treatments. Does he have Cat Scratch or does he have Lymphoma? Do they perform surgery to remove the lymph gland under his neck (and risk facial paralysis) or do we wait for it to go away? (which it would do if it were only Cat Scratch). Happy ending, he only had Cat Scratch!

Om symbol: This is a charm I brought home from the Self Realization Fellowship in Encinidas (not Encinada). This is the Hindu symbol for the cosmic vibration of the Universe. It is yet another representation of spirituality, and one more perspective of belief.

Heart with rose quartz: An acquaintance I met (a friend of my son's girlfriend) gave me this charm for my birthday (I think). She also loaned me a larger pennant with three healing stones on it. I wore that pennant every day throughout my chemotherapy treatments. Who am I to deny the healing powers of such stones. I'll take any form of healing I can get!

Pope cross: To learn the story behind this cross, please read update #9—Cathy Shares Reply. This is the charm that began my charm bracelet, and thus my charmed journey.

Peace symbol: The war with Iraq was ongoing through my treatments. As the mother of a son who has 5 friends fighting over there, this represents how I feel about this war.

Graduation cap & diploma: My son Paul graduated from high school 3 months after my last radiation treatment. His was not an easy year. I did my best to let him enjoy his senior year as much as possible without carrying the burden of a mother with cancer. I can't even begin to tell you how proud I am of this fine young man. Words are inadequate.

Celtic knot pattern: I already had this charm. I bought it years before at the Scottish Games. I added it to this bracelet for two reasons; 1. to remember the Scottish Games I attended, rolling around in the wheelchair and 2. to add a third charm to the bracelet (it looked quite sparse at first with just the cross and the Star of David on it).

Butterfly: This charm was given to me by my guardian angels at work. When all my treatments were done, they took me out to lunch and presented me with this charm for my bracelet to symbolize my "freedom" from treatment. I hope everyone has the chance to work with a group of people who feel like family (yet bicker less).

Top Right

Buddha: My friend Sue traveled to Bali while I was going through treatments, and hearing about my charm bracelet, brought me home this one to add to the collection. It adds to the world religions' symbolism I wanted to wear. It also reminds me of the wonderful "survivor" party that Sue and Pam gave me when I was done with my treatments.

Catherine's cross: I always tear up when I think of this gift. I have known Catherine for almost 15 years. Although we only work together on disability events a few times a year, we are quite fond of each other. She is an incredible woman. Catherine uses a wheelchair because of her long struggle with juvenile rheumatoid arthritis. I'll never forget the day we had lunch and she presented me with this cross to add to my bracelet. She shared with me the story of her hospitalization for several years during her teens. Her favorite nurse gave her this cross to remember her when she left. Catherine gave that very cross to me that day at lunch (are you crying yet? I still do when I see it on my bracelet.).

Celtic cross: I have three ear piercings, one in my left ear and two in my right ear. In the "extra" hole in my right ear I wore this cross from the day of surgery until my treatments were complete. Just another added form of protection. The last time I saw the matching cross to this set, it was in the ear of my dear Fedj somewhere in Los Angeles.

Computer: If you haven't figured it out already, this charm represents the writing of my updates, and my new-found love of writing. It also represents my new Dell computer and the patience I have learned while working with a PC (I am a Macintosh convert. Not by choice, by necessity).

Sun: We refer to our home in Paradise as "Casa del Sol" (house of the sun for those of you who flunked Spanish). I also like to think of it as "Casa del Soul" or "Soul Asylum"(asylum is a fitting word for crazy people like us). We have sun symbols hanging all over the inside and outside of the house, and on pots and other decorations. This charm symbolizes my new home which helped nurture me through my recovery.

Runner: This charm represents the American Cancer Society's Relay for Life events I performed for in Tracy and Lodi. I prepared a 2-minute dance/narration tribute to the fundraisers who gave so much time and energy to gather donations for research to find a cure. Preparing for these events gave me a dance focus to begin moving again and jump start my creative juices.

Hammer: One guess....that's right. The house remodeling! Very good.

Little man: This charm is the only thing I could find that looked like a man (except the runner). This represents Michael (Cupcake) and the time we spent together before he lost his battle to colon cancer. I will never forget him, his smile, his laugh. Sometimes God takes the good ones away from us, so heaven will be a little brighter.

Angel: I purchased this charm at the Scottish Games this year. It seemed fitting.

Elephant in costume: It may be hard to see, but this elephant is wearing a costume that closely resembles the pattern of my dance costume I made while going through treatments. It also represents how I felt when I wore my dance costume, having gained all that weight from chemotherapy.

Arm: Who would have ever thought I would find a charm of an arm?! This is my "Hope I don't get Lymphodema" charm. So far, so good.

My garden sign: This little wooden sign with the words "my garden" popping out of the flowers reminds me of the days I spent recovering, sitting in our garden of Eden in Paradise. Being surrounded by nature, watching the squirrels and birds, smelling the flowers, all these aspects of our garden helped me heal.

Circle clasp: In the jewelry business, these types of clasps are called "findings." On one of our trips to Encinitas (not Encinada) I was fortunate to hook up with a friend from my past who recently moved from Texas to Newport Beach California. She was the producer of a televised sign language class I did almost 20 years ago. I hadn't seen her in at least 5 years. She and her husband are now in the Venetian glass bead business and they gave me some beautiful jewelry, including this finding (top straight piece fits into the bottom circle piece). Her story of how they "found" their new calling to start this bead business reminds me of how I have "found" my new calling as a writer and cancer campaigner. It seems fitting that the clasp on this bracelet be a "finding."

Epilogue

At the time this book is printed it has now been 5 years since my cancer diagnosis. That magic number "5 years" is what cancer survivors dream to attain. It gives us some statistically based sense of hope that we can put this all behind us and move on. Today I continue to be cancer free.

For years I continued to participate in cancer fundraising activities. I created a wonderful character Polly Polyp for my employer's annual Cancer Awareness Campaign and with my parent's help designed this costume to bring her to life. Polly has also made appearances at Relay for Life and the Surviving Beautifully Fashion Show events.

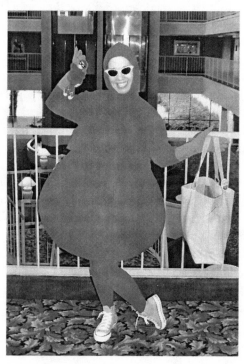

Polly Polyp educates audiences about preventing colon cancer.

The original epilogue that I wrote for this book was written over 3 years ago. It was the "Happily Ever After" ending to my cancer story with a picture of my wedding on the beach with Charlie. Although my marriage to Charlie lasted less than 3 years, I still consider my life to be Happily Ever After. Perhaps it was the return of previous challenges that Charlie and I had before my cancer diagnosis, perhaps it was the emotional instability that comes with taking Tamoxifen, perhaps it was a combination of both that led to the end of our marriage.

Two years ago my mother, my rock of Gibraltar, received the diagnosis that her cancer had returned after 20 years in remission. God and the medical professionals gave her 20 extra years and in her last year of life she was able to celebrate her 50th wedding anniversary and the love of her final grandchild. As I lay in bed holding her, singing her a lullaby as she took her last breath, I suddenly saw everything so vividly clear.

The support and love of people in our lives does not die when they do. Even when our dreams are dashed, we find new dreams to guide us. When infectious enthusiasm gives way to realistic questioning of the meaning of life, an under current of peace and gratitude sustains me.

Once my life returned to "normal" and I no longer felt the high that came from recent survivorship, all of the ongoing struggles of everday life returned and I found myself facing challenges with my old paradigm. I worked for over two years with a life coach who helped me get back on track (I highly recommend Dabbie and she can be reached at dbcoaching@earhlink.net). Preparing this manuscript for publication reminds me of my path and rekindles my desire to thrive. I have returned to the awareness and insight that I learned during my cancer journey. I continue to grow spiritually through reading and experiencing the teachings of others I seek to learn from. My life is still a *Cancer Dance;* from MRI to mammogram, one step at a time, I carefully choreograph each move for optimum life span and life joy.

The most valuable lesson my cancer taught me is that pain is inevitable and misery is optional. My gift to you is the recommendation…

Live…Breathe…Create…….DANCE!